Oxford Handbook
of Diabetes Nursing

Published and forthcoming Oxford Handbooks in Nursing

Oxford Handbook of Adult Nursing 3e
Oxford Handbook of Cancer Nursing 2e
Oxford Handbook of Cardiac Nursing 3e
Oxford Handbook of Children's and Young People's Nursing 2e
Oxford Handbook of Clinical Skills for Children's and Young People's Nursing
Oxford Handbook of Critical Care Nursing 2e
Oxford Handbook of Dental Nursing
Oxford Handbook of Diabetes Nursing 2e
Oxford Handbook of Emergency Nursing 3e
Oxford Handbook of Gastrointestinal Nursing 2e
Oxford Handbook of Learning and Intellectual Disability Nursing 2e
Oxford Handbook of Mental Health Nursing 2e
Oxford Handbook of Midwifery 4e
Oxford Handbook of Musculoskeletal Nursing 2e
Oxford Handbook of Neuroscience Nursing 2e
Oxford Handbook of Perioperative Practice 2e
Oxford Handbook of Prescribing for Nurses and Allied Health Professionals 3e
Oxford Handbook of Primary Care and Community Nursing 3e
Oxford Handbook of Respiratory Nursing 2e
Oxford Handbook of Surgical Nursing
Oxford Handbook of Trauma and Orthopaedic Nursing 2e
Oxford Handbook of Women's Health Nursing 2e

Oxford Handbook of Diabetes Nursing

SECOND EDITION

EDITED BY

Nicola Milne

Queen's Nurse
Primary Care Diabetes Specialist Nurse
Northenden Group Practice
Manchester, UK

Teffy Thomas

Advanced Clinical Practitioner in Diabetes
Clinical Lead for Inpatient Diabetes Team
Diabetes, Endocrine and Metabolism Centre
Manchester Royal Infirmary
Manchester Foundation Trust
Manchester, UK

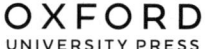

OXFORD
UNIVERSITY PRESS

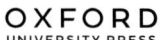

Great Clarendon Street, Oxford, OX2 6DP,
United Kingdom

Oxford University Press is a department of the University of Oxford.
It furthers the University's objective of excellence in research, scholarship,
and education by publishing worldwide. Oxford is a registered trade mark of
Oxford University Press in the UK and in certain other countries

First Edition published in 2009
Second Edition published in 2025

Published in the United States of America by Oxford University Press
198 Madison Avenue, New York, NY 10016, United States of America

British Library Cataloguing in Publication Data
Data available

Library of Congress Control Number: 2024945309

ISBN 978–0–19–883184–6

DOI: 10.1093/med/9780198831846.001.0001

Printed and bound in China by
C&C Offset Printing Co., Ltd.

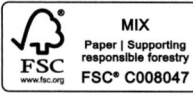

The manufacturer's authorised representative in the
EU for product safety is Oxford University Press
España S.A. of El Parque Empresarial San Fernando
de Henares, Avenida de Castilla, 2 – 28830 Madrid
(www.oup.es/en or product.safety@oup.com). OUP
España S.A. also acts as importer into Spain of
products made by the manufacturer.

Foreword

The first edition of this book was published in 2009, reflecting diabetes care and management at that time.

Since then, the prevalence of diabetes has increased significantly. It is estimated that more than 5.6 million people in the UK are now living with diabetes. Approximately 8% are people with type 1 diabetes, 92% are people with type 2 diabetes and the remaining 2% is associated with other causes for diabetes. The NHS spends at least £10 billion a year on diabetes which is about 10% of its entire budget. Almost 80% of the money the NHS spends on diabetes is on treating complications. In some hospitals over a quarter of beds are taken by people with diabetes (*Diabetes UK 2024*).[1]

With increasing prevalences of diabetes reflected worldwide, the majority, if not all working health care professionals will care for someone with diabetes almost every working day. The dynamic and ever-evolving nature of diabetes care presents both challenges and opportunities to improve outcomes for people living with diabetes; from understanding the pathophysiology of diabetes, to preventing and managing complications and providing education, every aspect of diabetes care requires an individualized approach, guided by evidence-based practice.

The role of the nurse has never been more critical in shaping the course and outcomes in diabetes care and it is therefore essential that the clinical skills and competences of nurses are enhanced to deliver appropriate levels of care within primary, community, and secondary care settings.

The Oxford Handbook of Diabetes Nursing serves as both a practical guide and insightful resource for nurses working with people with diabetes whether you are just starting your nursing career, have years of experience or undertaking post graduate study in diabetes.

As healthcare continues to evolve, the demand for specialized knowledge and skill in managing chronic conditions like diabetes will only increase.

I am confident that this book, available in both hard and online copies, will be a valuable resource in providing nurses and other health care professionals with the knowledge and tools they need to enhance their diabetes understanding and skills so to deliver excellence in diabetes nursing and make a meaningful difference to the lives of people living with diabetes.

Lorraine Avery
Diabetes Nurse Specialist: Clinical lead diabetes Brunel PCN

Reference

1. Hex N, MacDonald R, Pocock J, et al. Estimation of the direct health and indirect societal costs of diabetes in the UK using a cost of illness model. *Diabetic Medicine* 2024;41:e15326. doi:10.1111/dme.15326

Preface

The Oxford Book of Diabetes Nursing was first published in 2009, and this second edition the pocket-sized handbook serves as an update to support knowledge for contemporaneous, holistic, and gold standards of care in diabetes.

Within this addition, again written by experienced diabetes practitioners, the focus is on diabetes care across all settings to include primary, community, and inpatient diabetes care.

There is a wealth of evidenced based, practical guidance delivered in an easy-to-read format.

New chapters include psychological considerations in caring for people living with diabetes, female health, the perioperative management of diabetes and technology for insulin delivery and glucose monitoring.

Within other chapters there is inclusion of areas which have developed over more recent years such as type 2 diabetes prevention, the remission of type 2 diabetes, cardio-renal protection, frailty assessment, and multiple long-term conditions review. There is also a comprehensive section on insulin, to include advice on insulin types, devices, safety, and best practice injection technique.

Many of the chapters have associated case studies to support enhanced learning.

Throughout the book there is a focus on potential health inequalities, the importance of individualized care and how underserved communities can best be supported.

As with all publications, as evidence changes, it is important for the reader to ensure awareness of their local/national contemporaneous guidelines where relevant.

We express gratitude to all our contributors for sharing their time and expertise to include our reviewers for their care and rigor.

As we look to effective diabetes care delivery by the whole multidisciplinary team, we feel that this handbook is well equipped in providing high standards of education, guidance, and signposting for all healthcare professionals.

Acknowledgements

As co-editors, Teffy and I would like to acknowledge our colleagues who have willingly contributed their time and expertise in writing some of the chapters for the book and those who have reviewed the book content for us.

Personally, I would like to thank 'both' my families:

To the wonderful one at home, for encouragement, support and providing 'time'.

To the one in my working life, filled with amazing diabetes professionals who work with such dedication in advancing care. You all know who you are.

'Always have belief and shine bright'.

Nicola Milne

I would like to greatly thank my co-editor Nicki for giving me this wonderful opportunity and helping me throughout the book writing journey.

Thanks also goes to all those people with diabetes who have inspired and helped me learn more about diabetes.

Finally, I would like to deeply thank my friends and family, especially my daughter Anna, whose unwavering support, love and encouragement made this book possible.

Teffy Thomas

Contents

Contributors

Beverley Bostock, PgDip (Diabetes), MSc (Respiratory Care), MA (Med Ethics and Law), QN
Advanced Nurse Practitioner
Asthma Lead, Association of Respiratory Nurses
Primary Care Respiratory Society Executive Committee Member
Primary Care Cardiovascular Society Council Member
Editor in Chief, Practice Nurse Journal
Independent Training Consultant
Hereford, UK
Chapter 10: Macrovascular complications of diabetes: prevention and management

Alyson Chapman, RGN, BSc, MSc
DAFNE Educator
Diabetes Specialist Nurse
Manchester Diabetes, Endocrine and Metabolism Centre
Manchester Royal Infirmary
Manchester Foundation Trust
Manchester, UK
Chapter 6: Continuous subcutaneous insulin infusion

Jane Diggle, BSc (Hons) Nursing, RGN, NMP
Specialist Diabetes Nurse Practitioner
College Lane Surgery, West Yorkshire
Editor-in-Chief Diabetes & Primary Care
Committee member & Former Co Vice-Chair of The Primary Care Diabetes and Obesity Society
Chapter 5: Insulin use in diabetes
Chapter 17: Other important areas of diabetes care

Su Down, RGN, MSc, NMP
Nurse Consultant—Diabetes
Somerset NHS Foundation Trust
Editor-in-Chief Journal Diabetes Nursing
Committee member of The Primary Care Diabetes and Obesity Society
Somerset, UK
Chapter 1: Classification of diabetes
Chapter 14: Female health and diabetes

Jiney Edward, RGN, BSc (Hons), MSc (Advanced Clinical Practice)
Advanced Clinical Practitioner
Manchester Royal Eye Hospital
Manchester Foundation Trust
Manchester, UK
Chapter 11: Microvascular complications of diabetes: prevention and management

Agnieszka Graja, MSc, PGCert, RGN
Diabetes Specialist Nurse
Dorset County Hospital NHS Foundation Trust
Dorset, UK
Chapter 1: Classification of diabetes

Sarah Gregory, RGN, BSc (Hons), MSc (Diabetes)
Diabetes Specialist Nurse (Primary Care)
Northdown Surgery and Mocketts Wood Surgery
Diabetes UK Clinical Champion
Chapter 13: The older person with diabetes

Kelly Hayes, BSc (Podiatry), MSc (Podiatry)
Advanced Podiatrist—High Risk Care
Manchester Foundation Trust

Manchester Royal Infirmary
Manchester, UK
Chapter 11: Microvascular complications of diabetes: prevention and management

Jayne Hince, RN, BSc (Hons) Community Health

Diabetes Specialist Nurse/Antenatal
Manchester Diabetes, Endocrine and Metabolic Centre
Manchester Foundation Trust
Manchester, UK
Chapter 15: Diabetes in pregnancy

Madeline Little, BSc (Hons) (Dietetics), PGCert (Sports and Exercise Nutrition)

Team Lead Diabetes Dietitian
Manchester Diabetes, Endocrinology and Metabolism Centre
Peter Mount Building
Manchester Royal Infirmary
Manchester Foundation Trust
Manchester, UK
Chapter 4: Dietary management of diabetes

Nicola Milne, RGN, RM,

Queen's Nurse
Primary Care Diabetes Specialist Nurse
Northenden Group Practice,
Diabetes Specialist Nurse Clinical Lead for Greater Manchester and East Cheshire SCN
Manchester
Co-Vice Chair the Primary Care Diabetes and Obesity Society
Diabetes UK Clinical Champion
Manchester, UK
Chapter 1: Classification of diabetes
Chapter 2: Type 2 diabetes
Chapter 7: Assessment of glycaemia and management of non-urgent hyperglycaemia
Chapter 9: Ongoing care for people with diabetes

Chapter 10: Macrovascular complications of diabetes: prevention and management
Chapter 11: Microvascular complications of diabetes: prevention and management
Chapter 12: Acute complications of diabetes
Chapter 14: Female health and diabetes
Chapter 17: Other important areas of diabetes care
Chapter 18: Diabetes care delivery

Rose Stewart

Seicolegydd Clinigol Ymgynghorol | Consultant Clinical Psychologist
Arweinydd Seicoleg Diabetes | Diabetes Psychology Lead
Chair—UK Diabetes Psychology Network
Diabetes UK Clinical Champion
Wales, UK
Chapter 8: Psychological issues in people living with diabetes

Teffy Thomas, RGN, BSc (Hons), MSc (Advanced Clinical Practice)

Advanced Clinical Practitioner in Diabetes
Clinical Lead for Inpatient Diabetes Team
Diabetes, Endocrinology and Metabolism Centre
Manchester Royal Infirmary
Manchester Foundation Trust
Manchester, UK
Chapter 3: Type 1 diabetes
Chapter 11: Microvascular complications of diabetes: prevention and management
Chapter 12: Acute complications of diabetes
Chapter 16: Perioperative management of diabetes
Chapter 18: Diabetes care delivery

Reviewers:

Vicki Alabraba, MSc Diabetes Practice, RN
Education & Research Associate |
Diabetes Specialist Nurse
EDEN Team, Leicester
Diabetes Centre
Leicester, UK

Naresh Kanumilli, MB, BS, MRCGP, DFFP
Community Diabetes Consultant—
Manchester University
Foundation Trust
Chair of The Primary Diabetes and
Obesity Society
Diabetes UK Clinical Champion
Clinical Network Lead for
Diabetes—Greater Manchester &
East Cheshire
Manchester, UK

Abbreviations

AAC	Accelerated Access Collaborative		DASH	Dietary Approach to Stop Hypertension
ABPI	ankle–brachial pressure index		DCAP	Diabetes Care Accreditation Programme
ABPM	ambulatory blood pressure monitoring		DCCT	Diabetes Control and Complications Trial
ACEi	angiotensin-converting enzyme inhibitor		DDS	Diabetes Distress Scale
ACR	albumin:creatinine ratio		DEPS-R	Disordered Eating Problem Survey—revised
ADA	American Diabetes Association		DiaST	Diabetes Support Team
ADHD	attention-deficit/hyperactivity disorder		DiRECT	Diabetes Remission Clinical Trial
AKI	acute kidney injury		DKA	diabetic ketoacidosis
ARB	angiotensin receptor blocker		DPP-4	dipeptidyl peptidase type 4
ARF	acute renal failure		DR	diabetic retinopathy
ASCVD	atherosclerotic cardiovascular disease		DSM	diabetes specialist midwife
			DSN	diabetes specialist nurse
BG	blood glucose		DVLA	Driver and Vehicle Licensing Agency
BMI	body mass index			
BNF	British National Formulary		EASD	European Association for the Study of Diabetes
BP	blood pressure			
BPT	Best Practice Tariff		ED	emergency department; erectile dysfunction
CANVAS	Canagliflozin Cardiovascular Assessment Study		EDKA	euglycaemic diabetic ketoacidosis
CBG	capillary blood glucose		eFI	Electronic Frailty Index
CBGM	capillary blood glucose monitoring		eGFR	estimated glomerular filtration rate
CGM	continuous glucose monitoring		EMPA-REG	Empagliflozin, Cardiovascular Outcome Event Trial in Type 2 Diabetes Mellitus Patients
CHD	coronary heart disease			
CKD	chronic kidney disease			
CNS	central nervous system		EOT2D	early-onset type 2 diabetes
COVID-19	coronavirus disease 2019		EPIDIAR	Epidemiology of Diabetes and Ramadan (study)
CPOC	Centre for Perioperative Care			
CSII	continuous subcutaneous insulin infusion		ESC	European Society of Cardiology
CSME	clinically significant macular oedema		ESRD	end-stage renal disease
			FDA	Food and Drug administration
CV	cardiovascular		FH	familial hypercholesterolaemia
CVD	cardiovascular disease		FINDRISC	Finnish Diabetes Risk Score
CVOT	cardiovascular outcomes trial		FSD	female sexual dysfunction
DAFNE	Dose Adjustment for Normal Eating		FSFI	Female Sexual Function Index
			GAD	glutamic acid decarboxylase
DAN	diabetic autonomic neuropathy		GDM	gestational diabetes mellitus
			GI	glycaemic index

GIP	glucose-dependent insulinotropic polypeptide
GIRFT	Getting It Right First Time
GLP-1	glucagon-like peptide 1
GLP-1RA	glucagon-like peptide 1 receptor agonist
GP	general practitioner
HbA1c	glycated haemoglobin
HBPM	home blood pressure monitoring
HCL	hybrid closed loop
HCP	health care professional
HDL	high-density lipoprotein
HDL-C	high-density lipoprotein cholesterol
HF	heart failure
HFpEF	heart failure with preserved ejection fraction
HFrEF	heart failure with reduced ejection fraction
HHF	hospitalizations for heart failure
HHS	hyperosmolar hyperglycaemic state
HIV	human immunodeficiency virus
HLA	human leucocyte antigen
HONK	hyperosmolar non-ketotic (coma)
HRT	hormonal replacement therapy
IA-2	insulinoma antigen 2
IAPT	Improving Access to Psychological Therapies
ICA	islet cell cytoplasmic autoantibodies
ICB	Integrated Care Board
iDEAL	Insights for Diabetes Excellence, Access and Learning
IDF	International Diabetes Federation
IFCC	International Federation of Clinical Chemistry
IP3D	Improving the Perioperative Pathway for Patients with Diabetes
isCGM	intermittently scanned continuous glucose monitoring
IVI	intravitreal injection
IWGDF	International Working Group on the Diabetic Foot
JBDS	Joint British Diabetes Societies

KDIGO	Kidney Disease: Improving Global Outcomes
KFRE	Kidney Failure Risk Equation
KPD	ketosis-prone type 2 diabetes
LADA	latent autoimmune diabetes in adults
LARC	long-acting reversible contraception
LDL	low-density lipoprotein
LDL-C	low-density lipoprotein cholesterol
LOPS	loss of protective sensation
MACE	major all-cause cardiac events major adverse cardiovascular events
MDI	multiple daily injection; multiple-dose insulin
MDT	multidisciplinary team
MHRA	Medicines and Healthcare products Regulatory Agency
MI	myocardial infarction
MIDD	maternally inherited diabetes and deafness
MMC	maternal medicine clinic
MODY	maturity-onset diabetes of the young
NaDIA	National Diabetes Inpatient Audit
NCEPOD	National Confidential Enquiry into Patient Outcome and Death
NDH	non-diabetic hyperglycaemia
NDISA	National Diabetes Inpatient Safety Audit
NHS	National Health Service
NICE	National Institute for Health and Care Excellence
NPDA	National Pregnancy in Diabetes Audit
NPDR	non-proliferative diabetic retinopathy
NPID	National Diabetes in Pregnancy Audit
NSAID	non-steroidal anti-inflammatory drug
OCT	optical coherence tomography
OGTT	oral glucose tolerance test
PAD	peripheral arterial disease
PAID	Problem Areas In Diabetes Questionnaire
PCN	primary care network
PCOS	polycystic ovary syndrome

PDE5	phosphodiesterase 5	T1D	type 1 diabetes
PDR	proliferative diabetic retinopathy	T2D	type 2 diabetes
		T1DE	type 1 disordered eating
Periop DSN	perioperative diabetes specialist nurse	TDR	total diet replacement
		TGA	Therapeutic Goods Administration
PERT	pancreatic enzyme replacement therapy	TIR	time in range
PNDM	permanent neonatal diabetes	TNDM	transient neonatal diabetes
PRP	panretinal photocoagulation	UKMEC	UK Medical Eligibility Criteria
RAS	renin–angiotensin system	UKPDS	United Kingdom Prospective Diabetes Study
rDNA	recombinant DNA		
rtCGM	real-time continuous glucose monitoring	VEGF	vascular endothelial growth factor
SARS-CoV-2	severe acute respiratory syndrome coronavirus 2	VLED	very low-energy diet
		VRII	variable-rate insulin infusion
SDE	structured diabetes education	VRIII	variable-rate intravenous insulin infusion
SGLT2	sodium–glucose cotransporter 2		
		VTDR	vision-threatening diabetic retinopathy
SMI	severe mental health illness		
SMPC	summary of product characteristics	WHO	World Health Organization
		ZnT8	zinc transporter isoform 8
TA	Technology Appraisal		
TC	total cholesterol		

Classification of diabetes

Background

Diabetes has existed as long as mankind. Hieroglyphs in the Egyptian pyramids and ancient Asian Sanskrit writings describe the symptoms only too familiar today (see ➲ Chapters 2 and 3).

Before the discovery and purification of insulin for clinical use in the 1920s by a group of researchers in Toronto to include Frederick Banting, JJR Macleod, Charles Best, and James Collip, the only treatment for diabetes was a near-starvation diet until the inevitability of death.

Globally, at the time of writing, >1 in 10 adults are living with diabetes, which the International Diabetes Federation (IDF) in their *Diabetes Atlas* in 2021[1] described as 'a major health issue'.

In the UK, it is now estimated that for the first time, 5 million (4.3 million registered and an estimated 850,000 yet undiagnosed) people are living with diabetes, which equates to around 1 in 14 people.[2] Diabetes registrations have almost doubled in the last 15 years. This rise in diabetes prevalence is expected to continue, with 5.5 million people expected to have diabetes in the UK by 2030.[3]

There is evidence of a significant rise in the number of younger persons living with type 2 diabetes (T2D), with those under 40 years now accounting for 4% of the UK T2D population.[4]

Of important consideration is that 850,000 persons are currently thought to have T2D but have yet to be diagnosed, and 13 million people are considered to be at risk of developing T2D. This serves to underline the need for appropriate screening and T2D prevention strategies.

The various types of diabetes will be described later in the chapter, but typically 90% of diabetes cases are due to T2D, 8% due to type 1 diabetes (T1D), and 2% due to less common causes.

All types of diabetes have the potential for hyperglycaemic and cardiometabolic states, which can lead to both micro- and macrovascular complications. These include cardiovascular disease, neuropathy, nephropathy, retinopathy, and heart failure. The direct costs of diabetes in 2021/22 for the UK were estimated at £10.7 billion, of which just over 40% were related to diagnosis and treatment, with the rest relating to excess costs of complications. Indirect costs were estimated at £3.3 billion.[5] In the UK, there are estimated to be 700 premature deaths a week due to the physical effects of diabetes.[6]

Diabetes can also affect a person's emotional and mental well-being with, for example, a 50% ↑ risk for a person to experience depression and to be more likely to have depression for longer and more frequently.[7]

References

1. International Diabetes Federation (2021). *Diabetes Atlas*, 10th edition. Available at: ℜ https://diabetesatlas.org/idfawp/resource-files/2021/07/IDF_Atlas_10th_Edition_2021.pdf
2. Diabetes UK (2022). *Diabetes is serious*. Available at: ℜ https://diabetes-resources-production.s3.eu-west-1.amazonaws.com/resources-s3/public/2022-04/Diabetes%20is%20Serious%20Report%20Digital_0.pdf
3. Diabetes UK (2023). *Number of people living with diabetes in the UK tops 5 million for the first time*. Available at: ℜ www.diabetes.org.uk/about_us/news/number-people-living-diabetes-uk-tops-5-million-first-time

4. NHS England (2023). *National Diabetes Audit 2021–22, young people with type 2 diabetes–overview*. Available at: ℘ https://digital.nhs.uk/data-and-information/publications/statistical/national-diabetes-audit-yt2/young-people-with-type-2-diabetes-2021-22

5. Hex N, MacDonald R, Pocock J, Uzdzinska B, Taylor M, Atkin M, Wild SH, Beba H, Jones R. Estimation of the direct health and indirect societal costs of diabetes in the UK using a cost of illness model. *Diabetic Medicine*. 2024;**41**(9):e15326. doi:10.1111/dme.15326. Epub 2024 Jun 18. PMID: 38890775.

6. NHS England (2019). *National Diabetes Audit–report 2 complications and mortality, 2017–18*. Available at: ℘ https://digital.nhs.uk/data-and-information/publications/statistical/national-diabetes-audit/report-2--complications-and-mortality-2017-18

7. Mommersteeg PMC, Herr R, Pouwer F, Holt RIG, Loerbroks A. The association between diabetes and an episode of depressive symptoms in the 2002 World Health Survey: an analysis of 231,797 individuals from 47 countries. *Diabetic Medicine*. 2013;**30**(6):208–14.

The pancreas: overview

The pancreas is an elongated, leaf-shaped organ, pinkish in colour, lying across the back of the abdomen behind the stomach. The head of the pancreas, the widest part, lies to the right-hand side in the curve of the first section of the small intestine, the duodenum.

The body of the pancreas, the tapered left-hand side, extends upward towards the spleen, ending in the tail section. The pancreatic duct runs along the whole length of the pancreas.

The pancreas is covered with a thin connective tissue capsule that extends inward, partitioning the gland into lobules. It is made up of two types of cells: *exocrine* and *endocrine* (see Fig. 1.1).

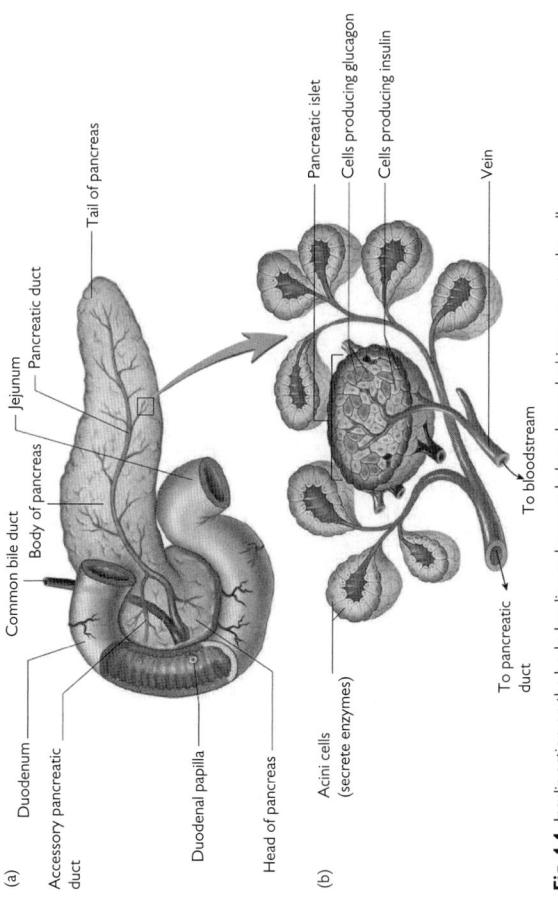

Fig. 1.1 Insulin action on the body. Insulin can be regarded as a key unlocking access to the cells.
Reproduced from Matthews D et al. (2008), *Diabetes*, with permission from Oxford University Press.

Exocrine functions of the pancreas

Exocrine anatomy

The majority of pancreatic cells are exocrine cells with their associated ducts. Embedded within this exocrine tissue are ~1 million grape-like cell clusters called acini. These are packed with membrane-bound secretory granules containing digestive enzymes, which pass through increasingly larger ducts until they flow into the main pancreatic duct and drain into the duodenum.

Exocrine physiology

Secretions from exocrine cells are vital to enable food to be completely digested, including protein, fat, and starch digestion.

Endocrine functions of the pancreas

Endocrine anatomy

There are ~1 million endocrine cells, called the islets of Langerhans, which comprise three major cell types:

- α-cells, which secrete glucagon
- β-cells, which produce insulin
- δ-cells, which secrete the hormone somatostatin (also produced by other endocrine cells).

The central part of each islet is occupied by β-cells, and α- and δ-cells cover this hub.

Secretion of insulin and glucagon is controlled by both parasympathetic and sympathetic neurons.

Endocrine physiology

The three hormones secreted by the endocrine tissue in the pancreas regulate the levels of glucose in the blood. They are:

- Insulin, which lowers blood glucose (BG) levels
- Glucagon, which promotes the release of glycogen from the liver, raising BG levels
- Somatostatin, which prevents the release of the other two hormones.

Insulin and glucagon are critical participants in glucose homeostasis and serve as acute regulators of blood glucose levels. Insulin is enormously important—a deficiency in insulin or deficit in insulin responsiveness leads to diabetes mellitus (see Fig. 1.2).

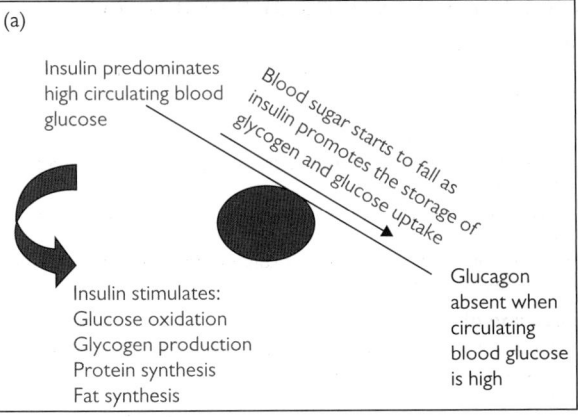

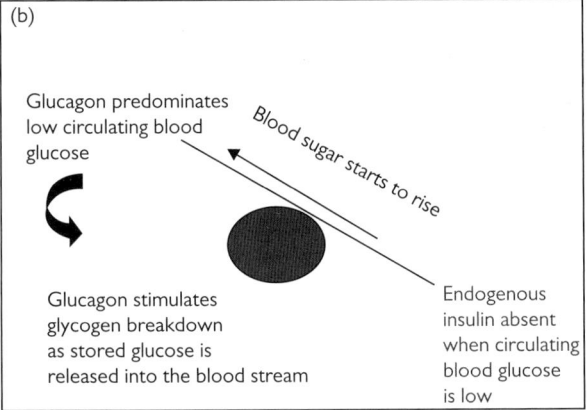

Fig. 1.2 Blood glucose regulation. (a) Fed state: postprandial. (b) Fasting state: preprandial or after having missed a meal.

Hormones

Insulin

- Synthesized in significant quantities only in β-cells in the pancreas.

Glucagon

This is the counter-regulatory hormone to insulin:
- Synthesized in α-cells in the pancreas.
- Secreted in response to:
  - Hypoglycaemia
  - Elevated blood levels of amino acids
  - Exercise.

When BG levels fall, glucagon is secreted. It facilitates the rise in BG levels in two ways:
- Glucagon stimulates the breakdown of glycogen stored in the liver.
- Glucagon activates hepatic gluconeogenesis (production of glucose).
  - Gluconeogenesis is the pathway by which non-hexose substrates, such as amino acids, are converted to glucose.
- Glucagon also has a minor effect of enhancing lipolysis of triglycerides in adipose tissue, which could be viewed as an additional means of conserving BG by providing fatty acid fuel to most cells.

Somatostatin

Secreted by a broad range of tissues, including the:
- Pancreas
- Intestinal tract
- Central nervous system (outside the hypothalamus).

Effects on the pancreas
- Inhibits secretion of insulin and glucagon.
- Suppresses pancreatic exocrine secretions.

Diabetes: an overview

Definition

In 2019, the World Health Organization (WHO)[1] described diabetes as 'a group of metabolic disorders characterised and identified by the presence of hyperglycemia in the absence of treatment'. Disorders in metabolism may be due to defects in insulin action and/or secretion and disturbances of carbohydrate, fat, and protein metabolism.

Classification of diabetes is important to ensure appropriate therapy and management.

Reference

1. International Diabetes Federation (2021). *Diabetes Atlas*, 10th edition. Available at: ℜ https:// diabetesatlas.org/idfawp/resource-files/2021/07/IDF_Atlas_10th_Edition_2021.pdf

Classification of diabetes

Type 1 diabetes

- Mostly autoimmune-mediated islet β-cell destruction, usually leading to absolute insulin deficiency.
- Associated with:
  - Pancreatic islet cell deficiency
  - Anti-glutamic acid decarboxylase (GAD) antibodies
  - Islet cell antibodies
  - Insulin antibodies.

People living with T1D can develop diabetic ketoacidosis (DKA), with elevated levels of hyperglycaemia (see ➲ Chapter 12, pp. 197–207). It commonly occurs in younger people but can present at any age. (See also ➲ Chapter 3.)

Type 2 diabetes

This comprises ~90% of all cases of diabetes and is classified according to various degrees of β-cell dysfunction and/or insulin resistance. It is commonly, but not always, associated with living with higher levels of visceral adiposity. It predominantly occurs in people over the age of 50 years, but cases are increasingly being seen in the younger population, including children. (See also ➲ Chapter 2.)

Hybrid forms of diabetes

Slowly evolving, immune-mediated diabetes of adults (also known as latent autoimmune diabetes in adults (LADA))

- May have features of metabolic syndrome but can be described as slowly evolving T1D in adults.
- Pancreatic function is retained for longer.

Key points for management
- Presence of any islet autoantibody (not necessarily GAD).
- Adult age of onset (>30 years).
- Often no requirement for insulin in the first 6–12 months of diagnosis.
- Initial misdiagnosis of T2D.
- Management is similar to that for T1D (see ⊃ Chapter 3).

Ketosis-prone type 2 diabetes (KPD)

- Initial presentation is usually with ketosis and severe insulin deficiency needing insulin replacement therapy.
- Later the person may no longer need insulin.
- The chance of a further ketotic episode occurring within 10 years is around 90%.
- No genetic markers or evidence of autoimmunity have been identified in KPD.
- Less common in populations of European origin.

Key points for management
- If no longer requiring insulin, the person will still need access to:
  - BG monitoring equipment to assess for any rising BG levels
  - A supply of in-date insulin if the need arises.
- May eventually be managed with lifestyle and/or oral therapies, but a sodium–glucose cotransporter 2 (SGLT2) inhibitor would be considered to be contraindicated due to history of ketosis (see ⊃ Chapter 2, Pharmacological management of hyperglycaemia, pp. 35–44).

Monogenic diabetes

Monogenic diabetes, often separated into neonatal diabetes and maturity-onset diabetes of the young (MODY), is a rare form of diabetes that results from mutations in a single gene. Unlike the more common types of diabetes (T1D and T2D), which are complex conditions influenced by multiple genes and environmental factors, monogenic diabetes is caused by a specific gene mutation.

Key points about monogenic diabetes

- Inheritance: monogenic diabetes is often inherited in an autosomal dominant pattern, meaning that a single copy of the mutated gene is sufficient to cause the condition. This means all children of an affected parent with monogenic diabetes have a 50% chance of inheriting the affected gene.
- Onset: it typically presents at a younger age (often before 25 years) and may be misdiagnosed as T1D or T2D.
- Genes: there are over 30 genes associated with monogenic diabetes, including *GCK*, *HNF1A*, *HNF4A*, and others.
- Treatment: can differ from that of T1D or T2D. Medications and lifestyle management may be tailored, based on the specific genetic mutation.
- Diagnosis: genetic testing is required to confirm a diagnosis of monogenic diabetes. This testing identifies the specific gene mutation responsible for the condition.

The likelihood of monogenic diabetes can be calculated via the probability calculator (available at: ℜ www.diabetesgenes.org/exeter-diabetes-app/ModyCalculator).

MODY affects 3.6% of those diagnosed below the age of 25 years, although it is initially misdiagnosed in around 77% of cases.

The three main features of MODY are:

- Diabetes often developing before the age of 25 years
- Diabetes presents in families from one generation to the next
- It may be treated by diet or tablets (typically sulfonylureas) and does not always need insulin treatment.

Monogenic diabetes encompasses several distinct subtypes, each associated with a specific gene mutation. The most common types of monogenic diabetes include:

- **GCK-MODY**: people with GCK-MODY have mildly elevated BG levels from birth, but it usually does not require treatment. It is often discovered incidentally and is not associated with complications.
- **HNF1A-MODY**: typically manifests as mild to moderate hyperglycaemia. It is often diagnosed in adolescence or early adulthood. Changes in the *HNF1A* gene cause diabetes by reducing the amount of insulin that is produced by the pancreas. HNF1A MODY is optimally treated with low doses of sulfonylureas initially.
- **HNF4A-MODY**: this subtype tends to develop diabetes in early adulthood, and it is often associated with macrosomia and neonatal hypoglycaemia. Recommended initial treatment would be sulfonylureas.

- ***HNF1B-MODY***: this subtype can present with a range of symptoms but is characterized by renal developmental abnormalities (typically cysts) and pancreatic insufficiency, often requiring treatment. Insulin is usually required.
- ***Neonatal diabetes***: diagnosed in the first 6 months of life. Common causes of neonatal diabetes include mutations in the potassium channel (KATP) genes *ABCC8* or *KCNJ11*; these subtypes can present with transient neonatal diabetes (TNDM) or permanent neonatal diabetes (PNDM). *KCNJ11* and *ABCC8* neonatal diabetes are best treated with high-dose sulfonylureas, but the other causes of neonatal diabetes require insulin treatment and may be associated with other features.
- ***Maternally inherited diabetes and deafness (MIDD)***: inherited from mothers—the genetic change is passed down from an affected mother to all her children. Deafness is bilateral and sensorineural and typically develops before diabetes. Men who have MIDD will not pass the condition on to their children, as all mitochondria are inherited from the mother. Insulin treatment is usually required within 2 years of diagnosis.

These subtypes of monogenic diabetes have different clinical presentations and require tailored treatment approaches. Genetic testing is necessary to confirm the specific subtype and guide management.

Genetic testing can help in the following ways:

- Diagnosis: it can confirm the presence of a monogenic form of diabetes, which may require different treatment approaches, compared with T1D or T2D.
- Risk assessment: genetic testing can determine the risk of passing on monogenic diabetes to offspring in families with the condition.
- Personalized treatment: identifying the specific genetic mutation can guide treatment choices, as some monogenic forms of diabetes respond better to certain medications.
- Family screening: genetic testing can be used to screen family members of affected individuals for the presence of the same mutation.

Criteria: eligibility criteria for genetic testing can be found at Diabetes Genes (available at: www.diabetesgenes.org)

The criteria for genetic testing apply to the proband (the first member of a family with diabetes to be tested). Once a genetic diagnosis of monogenic diabetes has been confirmed in the proband, other family members will be eligible for testing of the familial variant.

Further reading

Diabetes Genes. Available at: www.diabetesgenes.org

Exeter Clinical Laboratory. *Glutamic acid decarboxylase (GAD) antibodies*. Available at: www.exeterlaboratory.com/test/gad-antibodies/

Exeter Clinical Laboratory. *C-peptide creatinine ratio (UCPCR): urine*. Available at: www.exeterlaboratory.com/test/c-peptide-urine

Hattersley AT, Greeley SAW, Polak M, *et al*. ISPAD Clinical Practice Consensus Guidelines 2022: the diagnosis and management of monogenic diabetes in children and adolescents. *Pediatric Diabetes*. 2022;**23**;(8):1188–211.

Murphy R, Colclough K, Pollin TI, *et al*. The use of precision diagnostics for monogenic diabetes: a systematic review and expert opinion. *Communications Medicine*. 2023;**3**:136.

Diseases of exocrine function (often referred to as type 3c diabetes)

When diabetes occurs as a consequence of pancreatic damage, this is referred to as type 3c diabetes or pancreatic diabetes. It is a condition whereby there is structural damage to both exocrine and endocrine functionality of the pancreas and, as such, both elements will need treatment.

In Western populations, estimates vary, with one study suggesting that as many as 5–10% of all individuals with diabetes may have type 3c diabetes.[1]

It is frequently misclassified (often as T2D), and so prevalence is often underestimated in practice.

The most common conditions that cause type 3c diabetes are:
- Pancreatitis
- Pancreatectomy following trauma or surgery
- Neoplasia*
- Pancreatic destruction, for example, with cystic fibrosis
- Fibrocalculous pancreatopathy
- Haemochromatosis (a disease of iron storage).

Management of type 3c diabetes is often with insulin therapy and requires bespoke dietary advice. It often also requires enzyme replacement therapy to address the exocrine insufficiency. Careful advice and management of hypoglycaemia are important in type 3c diabetes, as pancreatic damage will also lead to loss of glucagon production.

Symptoms can be varied and vague, and include:
- Indigestion
- Abdominal and/or back pain
- Unexplained weight loss
- Nausea
- Loss of appetite
- Changes in bowel habit
- Jaundice—can be a symptom and would necessitate urgent referral.

Long-standing diabetes can also cause damage to the exocrine pancreas, and so people with established diabetes can also develop exocrine insufficiency and again will often require both insulin therapy and enzyme replacement therapy.

Diagnostic criteria

These may include:
- Pancreatic exocrine insufficiency (faecal elastase 1 testing)
- Pathological pancreatic imaging (endoscopic ultrasound/computed tomography or magnetic resonance imaging)
- Absence of type 1 diabetes-associated antibodies.

---

* Pancreatic cancer should be considered in new-onset diabetes in those aged over 60 years or in unstable diabetes in someone with T2D who has previously been stable. Risk factors include ↑ age, smoking, living with obesity, family history, pancreatitis, and diabetes.

Management

Diet and lifestyle
- High-soluble-fibre diet.
- Smoking cessation where appropriate.
- Avoidance of alcohol.
- Regular exercise.

Glycaemic management
- Insulin therapy is often required as β-cell failure can be rapid.
- Glucagon-like peptide 1 receptor agonists (GLP-1RAs) and dipeptidyl peptidase type 4 (DPP-4) inhibitors often need to be avoided due to caution in use in people with pancreatitis and potential undesirable weight loss with GLP-1RAs.
- Caution with SGLT2 inhibitors due to the increased risk of euglycaemic DKA and potential for undesirable weight loss.

Management of potential exocrine insufficiency
- Pancreatic enzyme replacement therapy (PERT) (e.g. Creon®, Nutrizym®, Pancrease®, Pancrex®) with meals.
- PERT can improve digestion of carbohydrates and ↑ BG levels; it may unmask diabetes in an individual with previously normal glycated haemoglobin (HbA1c).
- Vitamin D supplements if proven deficiency.
- Consider investigations for osteoporosis.

Reference

1. Morris D. Recognition and management of pancreatogenic (type 3c) diabetes. *Diabetes and Primary Care*. 2020;**22**:111–12.

Further reading

Pancreatic cancer UK. Available at: ℘ www.pancreaticcancer.org.uk

Diseases of the endocrine system

Cushing's syndrome

- ↑ production of glucose by the liver.
- ↑ insulin resistance at the peripheral tissue level.
- This results in ↑ BG levels.

Acromegaly

- Usually caused by a tumour in the pituitary gland, which causes excess growth hormone to be produced.
- Growth hormone ↑ insulin resistance.
- Over half of people with acromegaly have hyperinsulinaemia and glucose intolerance.

Phaeochromocytoma

- Excess adrenaline, a 'fight or flight' hormone is secreted, often because of a phaeochromocytoma, a tumour of the adrenal gland.
- Fight or flight response mobilizes glucose production to fuel the activity.
- Adrenaline acts on adrenoreceptors and ↑ insulin resistance.
- This inhibits insulin secretion and ↑ breakdown of fat and glycogen to glucose in the liver.

Glucagonoma

- Rare tumour of the pancreatic α-cells may ↑ glucagon levels, resulting in impaired glucose regulation.

Somatostatinoma

- Excess somatostatin secretion caused by a rare pancreatic tumour affecting pancreatic δ-cells.
- Inhibits insulin secretion and results in impaired glucose regulation.

Drug and chemical interactions

Many medications prescribed for specific purposes can inhibit the effect of insulin, acting as a trigger in those with a predisposition to diabetes.

Some hormones, when given in large doses, can impair the action of insulin (e.g. glucocorticoids, thyroid hormones).

It is important to check the British National Formulary (BNF) or individual summaries of product characteristics (SMPCs) for full details of drug interactions and contraindications.

Glucocorticoids

- Raise BG levels by counteracting some actions of insulin.
- Prolonged use of steroid therapy may lead to glucose intolerance and diabetes.

Principles of management of steroid-induced diabetes/hyperglycaemia

- Short courses of steroids resulting in minimal periods of hyperglycaemia may not warrant intervention.
- BG levels in most individuals can be predicted to rise ~4–8 hours following administration of oral steroids (sooner following administration of intravenous steroids).
- There may be a low impact on fasting BG levels, but significant effects on postprandial BG levels.
- The aim of management is to treat any hyperglycaemia whilst avoiding nocturnal/early morning hypoglycaemia.
- Screening for steroid-induced diabetes includes pre-commencement HbA1c and regular BG monitoring.
- If steroid-induced diabetes or steroid-induced hyperglycaemia, aim for BG targets of 6–10mmol/L or individualize based on frailty, comorbidities, and/or prognosis.
- Consider BG monitoring four times daily, and refresh diabetes education with the person and their families and/or carers.
- Metformin can be titrated to 1g twice daily.
- Gliclazide can be titrated to a maximum of 320mg daily, with up to 240mg taken in the morning.
- Basal NPH insulin can be given in the morning, and if BG levels remain uncontrolled, then prandial insulin may be added with appropriate meals (see ➲ Chapter 5, pp. 82–83).
- BG levels can return to normal as soon as 24 hours after stopping treatment: Always remember to review the de-escalation of medication with reducing steroid doses.

Immune checkpoint inhibitors

- Immunotherapies are cancer treatments that aim to stimulate the immune system to kill cancer cells. These include nivolumab and pembrolizumab.
- The stimulating effect can cause high BG levels.

Further reading

Joint British Diabetes Societies for Inpatient Care (2021). *Management of hyperglycaemia and steroid (glucocorticoid) therapy.* Available at: ℘ https://abcd.care/sites/abcd.care/files/site_uploads/JBDS_Guidelines_Archive/JBDS_08_Steroids_DM_Guideline_FINAL_28052021_Archive.pdf

Infections

Some viruses have been associated with β-cell destruction:
- Congenital rubella
- Cytomegalovirus.

Genetic syndromes

Genetic syndromes sometimes associated with diabetes include:
- Down syndrome
- Huntington's chorea
- Myotonic dystrophy
- Prader–Willi syndrome
- Turner's syndrome.

Post-transplant diabetes mellitus

This can occur following solid organ transplantation and is a risk factor for graft failure. In addition to standard risk factors for T2D, such as ethnicity and features of cardiometabolic syndrome, there are additional risk factors including immunosuppressive agents and potential infections.

Persons should be screened pre-transplantation for any possible established diabetes or related risk factors which should be managed appropriately.

Hyperglycaemia in the early post-operative period should be managed ideally with insulin therapy.

Once clinically stable, there may be an opportunity to reduce or stop insulin and to consider oral anti-hyperglycaemic medications.

Gestational diabetes

Gestational diabetes is diabetes that first appears in pregnancy and resolves post-partum. It is thought that placental hormones ↑ insulin resistance in the mother, leading to elevated BG levels.

- Usually identified in the second trimester of pregnancy.
- It commonly requires treatment with insulin for the duration of the pregnancy.
- BG levels return to normal following delivery.
- Usually occurs in subsequent pregnancies.
- Can often be a risk factor for T2D in later life (see ⊃ Chapter 2, p. 27).

(See ⊃ Chapter 15 on pregnancy and diabetes for further details, including risk factors, screening, and principles of management.)

Non-diabetic hyperglycaemia

Non-diabetic hyperglycaemia (NDH) is a predictor of ↑ risk of developing T2D.

Other terms which have been used to describe this include:
- Pre-diabetes
- Impaired glucose regulation
- Impaired fasting glucose
- Impaired glucose tolerance.

The National Institute for Health and Care Excellence (NICE) advocates for diagnosis based on HbA1c values of 42–47mmol/mol inclusively or fasting plasma glucose levels of 6.1–6.9mmol/L inclusively.

(For management of NDH, see ⊃ Chapter 2, pp. 28–29.)

Further reading

International Diabetes Federation (2021). *Diabetes Atlas*, 10th edition. Available at: ℛ https://diabet esatlas.org/idfawp/resource-files/2021/07/IDF_Atlas_10th_Edition_2021.pdf

World Health Organization (2019). *Classification of diabetes mellitus*. Available at: ℛ https://apps. who.int/iris/rest/bitstreams/1233344/retrieve

Diagnosis of, and diagnostic criteria for, diabetes

In 2011, the WHO[1] recommended that a diagnosis of diabetes could be made based on the values given in Box 1.1.

Signs and symptoms of diabetes

- Thirst.
- Polyuria (including nocturia).
- Weight loss.
- Infections (thrush, abscesses).
- Poor wound healing.
- Blurred vision.
- Tiredness and lethargy.

In the absence of symptoms, two abnormal results are required to make a diagnosis of T2D. Ideally, the same test should be used. When a HbA1c test is used, it should be repeated straight away to confirm the diagnosis (do not wait 3 months).[2]

Situations where a HbA1c test should *not* be used for diagnosis include:
- ALL children and young people
- Suspected T1D
- In acute illness (e.g. requiring hospital admission), post-severe trauma or cardiovascular event
- Taking medication that may cause rapid ↑ in BG levels (e.g. steroids, antipsychotics)
- Where a person has acute pancreatic damage, including pancreatic surgery
- Pregnancy
- End-stage renal disease
- In people being treated for human immunodeficiency virus (HIV) infection with certain antivirals.

BOX 1.1 Recommended metrics for the diagnosis of diabetes

- *Symptoms present (e.g. polyuria, thirst, unexplained weight loss):*
  - A single fasting plasma glucose ≥7.0mmol/L OR
  - A single random plasma glucose ≥11.1mmol/L OR
  - A HbA1c ≥48mmol/mol (6.5%)
- *No symptoms:*
  - A fasting plasma glucose ≥7.0mmol/L on two separate occasions OR
  - A random plasma glucose ≥11.1mmol/L on two separate occasions OR
  - A HbA1c ≥48mmol/mol (6.5%) on two separate occasions OR
  - A HbA1c ≥48mmol/mol AND a single elevated plasma glucose (fasting ≥7.0mmol/L or random ≥11.1mmol/L)

Interpret HbA1c results with caution if there is a condition causing abnormal red blood cell lifespan (e.g. anaemia, haemoglobinopathies).

Be aware that severe hyperglycaemia in people with an acute infection, trauma, and circulatory or other stress may be transitory and is not diagnostic of diabetes.

Other tests to support diagnosis

C-peptide
- C-peptide is a marker of endogenous insulin secretion from pancreatic β-cells.
- NICE[3] advises not to use routinely for diagnosis of T1D, but it may be useful in cases where differentiation between T1D and T2D is unclear.
- In established T1D, endogenous insulin secretion will be either very low or nil, with correspondingly low C-peptide levels.
- It should be performed with a paired plasma glucose level for appropriate interpretation.

Autoantibodies
- Can help to distinguish between autoimmune T1D and other forms of diabetes.
- Islet cell cytoplasmic autoantibodies (ICA) are present in 70–80% of T1D cases.
- GAD antibodies are present in 70–80% of T1D cases.
- Insulinoma-associated 2 antibodies are present in 60% of T1D cases.
- NICE[3] recommends measuring anti-GAD and anti-ICA antibodies in the diagnosis of T1D or LADA.

References

1. World Health Organization (2011). *Use of glycated haemoglobin (HbA1c) in the diagnosis of diabetes mellitus: abbreviated report of a WHO Consultation*. Available at: ℘ https://iris.who.int/bitstream/handle/10665/70523/WHO_NMH_CHP_CPM_11.1_eng.pdf
2. National Institute for Health and Care Excellence (2022). *Diabetes—type 2: When should I suspect type 2 diabetes in an adult?* Available at: ℘ https://cks.nice.org.uk/topics/diabetes-type-2/diagnosis/diagnosis-in-adults
3. National Institute for Health and Care Excellence (2015, updated 2022). *Type 1 diabetes in adults: diagnosis and management*. Available at: ℘ www.nice.org.uk/guidance/ng17/chapter/recommendations#diagnosis-and-early-care-plan

Type 2 diabetes

Incidence and epidemiology

Type 2 diabetes (T2D) is the most common form of diabetes, accounting for ~90% of people diagnosed with diabetes. The World Health Organization (WHO) estimated in 2021 that there were 537 million people globally living with diabetes and predicted a rise to 643 million by 2030.[1] This equates to somewhere in the region of 483 million people with T2D in 2021 and a predicted ↑ to just under 578 million by 2030.

It is important to be aware that up to 45% of diabetes cases remain undiagnosed, which is most predominantly incidences of T2D.

The increasing global prevalence of T2D is multifactorial. Factors include an ageing population, rising rates of obesity, and economic development to encompass urbanization, which generally leads to more sedentary lifestyles and ↑ consumption of foods related to obesity.

Reference

1. International Diabetes Federation (2021). *Diabetes Atlas*, 10th edition. Available at: ℘ https://diabetesatlas.org/idfawp/resource-files/2021/07/IDF_Atlas_10th_Edition_2021.pdf

Aetiology

T2D is associated with defects in the action and secretion of insulin.

Organs involved in T2D development include the pancreas (β- and α-cells), liver, skeletal muscle, kidneys, brain, small intestine, and adipose tissue.[1] Evolving data also suggest a role for adipokine dysregulation, abnormalities in gut microbiota, immune dysregulation, and inflammation as pathophysiological factors.[2]

A reduction in sensitivity to insulin (insulin resistance) generally precedes ↓ insulin production (see Fig. 2.1).

When the feedback loops between insulin action and secretion are dysfunctional, this leads to abnormal blood glucose levels.

Progression to type 2 diabetes

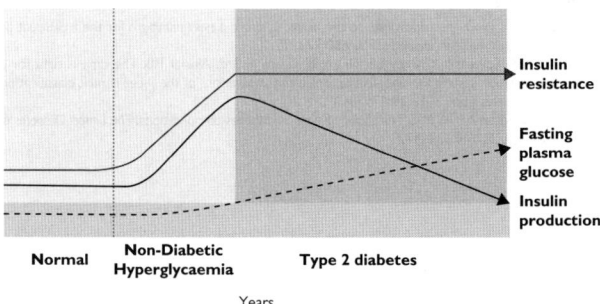

Fig. 2.1 Progression to type 2 diabetes.
Adapted from Bailey C. *British Journal of Cardiology* 2000;7(6):350–360; Defronzo RA, Ferranini E. *Diabetes Care* 1991;14(3):173–194.

Insulin resistance

This is associated with a group of clinical features known as 'metabolic syndrome'. These include abdominal obesity, reduced high-density lipoprotein (HDL) cholesterol levels, elevated triglyceride levels, and hypertension. It typically, but not always, reflects a sedentary lifestyle, overnutrition, and resultant excess adiposity, and is strongly associated with the development of endothelial dysfunction and atherosclerosis, resulting in ↑ risk of cardiovascular disease (CVD).

It leads to ↑ glucose production in the liver and ↓ glucose uptake in muscle and adipose tissue, resulting in raised circulating blood glucose levels and progression to T2D.

Hyperinsulinaemia

In the absence of lifestyle modification, insulin resistance develops and ↑ with the duration of diabetes. The immediate response of β-cells is to ↑ insulin production, which is known as hyperinsulinaemia. β-cell overwork eventually leads to β-cell failure and reduced production of insulin.

Complications of type 2 diabetes

Raised circulating glucose levels and the presence of associated metabolic conditions related to insulin resistance (e.g. hypertension, dyslipidaemia) ↑ the risk of micro- and macrovascular complications. These include microvascular-related conditions of retinopathy, nephropathy, neuropathy, erectile dysfunction, and autonomic dysfunction. Macrovascular complications include stroke, angina, myocardial infarction, and peripheral artery disease. All these potential complications will be discussed in greater detail in ➲ Chapters 9, 10, and 11.

Based on cohort studies, the relative risk of micro- and macrovascular disorders among people with diabetes is estimated to be at least 10–20 times higher for microvascular, and 2–4 times higher for macrovascular, complications, respectively, than in people without diabetes.[3]

References

1. Defronzo RA. From the triumvirate to the ominous octet: a new paradigm for the treatment of type 2 diabetes mellitus. *Diabetes*. 2009;**58**:773–95.
2. Schwartz SS, Epstein S, Corkey BE, Grant SF, Gavin JR 3rd, Aguilar RB. The time is right for a new classification system for diabetes: rationale and implications of the β-cell-centric classification schema. *Diabetes Care*. 2016;**39**:179–86.
3. Gregg EW, Sattar N, Ali MK. The changing face of diabetes complications. *The Lancet Diabetes & Endocrinology*. 2016;**4**:537–47.

Risk factors for developing type 2 diabetes

Non-modifiable

- Family history.
- Ethnicity.
- Older age.
- History of gestational diabetes.
- Low birthweight.
- Other endocrine disorders (e.g. thyrotoxicosis, Cushing's syndrome, acromegaly).
- Schizophrenia and severe mental illness.
- Need for certain hyperglycaemic medications (e.g. steroids, immunotherapy, some antipsychotic therapies).
- History of polycystic ovary syndrome.
- Certain HIV antiretroviral therapies.
- Post-transplantation therapies.

Modifiable risk factors

- Raised body mass index (BMI) based on ethnicity values.[1]
- Abdominal or central obesity, independent of BMI.
- Raised waist circumference or waist-to-hip ratio.
- Sedentary lifestyle.
- A diet with high-glycaemic index carbohydrates, and foods and drinks high in saturated fats, salt, and sugar.
- Cigarette smoking.
- Components of metabolic syndrome such as hypertension and dyslipidaemia.
- Presence or history of non-diabetic hyperglycaemia.
- Psychosocial stress and depression.
- Presence of periodontal disease.

Reference

1. Caleyachetty R, Barber TM, Ibrahim Mohammed N, *et al*. 2021 Ethnicity-specific BMI cutoffs for obesity based on type 2 diabetes risk in England: a population-based cohort study. *The Lancet Diabetes & Endocrinology*. 2021;**9**:419–26. Available at: ℘ www.thelancet.com/journals/landia/article/PIIS2213-8587(21)00088-7/fulltext#%20

Prevention of type 2 diabetes

Since 2000, the estimated global prevalence of diabetes in adults aged 20–79 years has more than tripled, from an estimated 151 million to 537 million.[1]

Much is driven by the rise in cases of T2D.

However, there is evidence from several major T2D prevention studies[2,3,4,5] that lifestyle/behavioural interventions can be effective in delaying, or indeed preventing, the onset of T2D and improving other associated cardiometabolic markers such as lipid levels and blood pressure.

With the number of persons with diabetes expected to rise to 783 million by 2045 without intervention,[1] it is important that we look globally, nationally, and locally at T2D strategies focused on modifiable risk factors.

Lifestyle advice the prevention of type 2 diabetes

- Diet and physical activity for weight loss where appropriate (see ➜ Lifestyle guidance, pp. 33–34).
- Smoking cessation where relevant.
- Promotion of mental and emotional well-being (see ➜ Chapter 8).
- Promotion of healthy sleeping patterns (see ➜ Lifestyle guidance, pp. 33–34).

Strategies the prevention of type 2 diabetes

- Identification of high-risk groups:
  - For cohorts thought to be at higher risk of developing T2D, see ➜ Risk factors for developing type 2 diabetes, p. 27.
  - Use of T2D risk assessment tools, such as Diabetes UK 'Know your Risk'[6] or the diabetes risk calculator 'FINDRISC' (Finnish Diabetes Risk Score),[7] to determine the level of risk.
  - Offer blood test screening to those identified at higher risk.
  - Keep a list of those at higher risk to include women with a history of gestational diabetes.
- *Low risk* (on risk score):
  - Advise the risk is currently low, but this could change in the future. Give appropriate lifestyle advice.
  - Offer referral/signposting to any applicable local or national services which may help in reducing risk (e.g. weight management services).
  - Reassess risk every 5 years.
- *Moderate risk* (moderate or high on risk score, but HbA1c <42mmol/mol or fasting glucose <5.5mmol/L):
  - Advise on the risk being moderate and look to specific lifestyle advice.
  - Offer referral/signposting to any applicable local or national support services which may help in reducing risk (e.g. weight management services).
  - Offer reassessment every 3 years.
- *High risk* (raised on risk score; HbA1c 42–47mmol/mol or fasting glucose 5.5–6.9mmol/L or history of previous gestational diabetes):
  - Explain that the risk of progression to T2D is high, but not inevitable (it is thought that 30–58% of persons will progress to T2D without intervention).[8]

- Advise that the risk can be reduced with lifestyle intervention.
- Reassess annually with appropriate advice.
- Refer to any available local or nationally commissioned diabetes prevention programme.

The *NHS England Diabetes Prevention Programme*[9] is an example of a nationally commissioned, evidence-based programme for people at high risk of developing T2D, providing tailored support to reduce risk through lifestyle changes.

It provides support over a minimum of 9 months to help people at high risk of T2D to improve their diet, ↑ physical activity, and achieve a healthy weight.

Other considerations

As T2D is a cardiometabolic condition, those at risk of progression will also benefit from assessment of blood pressure, lipid profiles, and cardiovascular and renal status (for greater detail on macro- and microvascular complications, respectively, see ➔ Chapter 10, ➔ Chapter 11).

References

1. International Diabetes Federation (2021). *Diabetes Atlas*, 10th edition. Available at: ℅ https://diabetesatlas.org/idfawp/resource-files/2021/07/IDF_Atlas_10th_Edition_2021.pdf
2. Knowler WC, Barrett-Connor E, Fowler SE, *et al.*; Diabetes Prevention Program Research Group. Reduction in the incidence of type 2 diabetes with lifestyle intervention or metformin. *New England Journal of Medicine*. 2002;**346**(6):393–403.
3. Lindström J, Ilanne-Parikka P, Peltonen M, *et al.*; Finnish Diabetes Prevention Study Group. Sustained reduction in the incidence of type 2 diabetes by lifestyle intervention: follow-up of the Finnish Diabetes Prevention Study. *The Lancet*. 2006;**368**(9548):1673–9.
4. Li G, Zhang P, Wang J, *et al.* Cardiovascular mortality, all-cause mortality, and diabetes incidence after lifestyle intervention for people with impaired glucose tolerance in the Da Qing Diabetes Prevention Study: a 23-year follow-up study. *The Lancet Diabetes & Endocrinol*. 2014;**2**(6):474–80.
5. Ramachandran A, Snehalatha C, Mary S, Mukesh B, Bhaskar AD, Vijay V; Indian Diabetes Prevention Programme (IDPP). The Indian Diabetes Prevention Programme shows that lifestyle modification and metformin prevent type 2 diabetes in Asian Indian subjects with impaired glucose tolerance (IDPP-1). *Diabetologia*. 2006;**49**(2):289–97.
6. Diabetes UK. Know Your Risk Score. Available at: ℅ https://riskscore.diabetes.org.uk/start
7. FINDRISC (Finnish Diabetes Risk Score). Available at: ℅ www.mdcalc.com/calc/4000/findrisc-finnish-diabetes-risk-score
8. Nichols GA, Hillier TA, Brown JB. Progression from newly acquired impaired fasting glucose to type 2 diabetes. *Diabetes Care*. 2007;**30**(2):228–33. Erratum in: *Diabetes Care*. 2008;**31**(12):2414.
9. NHS England. *NHS Diabetes Prevention Programme (NHS DPP). Preventing type 2 diabetes*. Available at: ℅ www.england.nhs.uk/diabetes/diabetes-prevention

Presentation of type 2 diabetes

T2D traditionally presented in middle age or later life. However, there is now a growing prevalence of cases in younger age groups to include children.

T2D onset is usually insidious and may go undiagnosed for several years. People may be diagnosed because of routine screening as part of health check programmes or cardiovascular reviews; thus, presentation is commonly without the classical symptoms of hyperglycaemia. However, this does not exclude a presentation of someone with osmotic symptoms such as tiredness, thirst, nocturia, and unintentional weight loss.

NB for anyone with significant unintentional weight loss over the age of 60 years, it is important to rule out any possibility of pancreatic neoplasia (see ⊃ Chapter 1).

T2D may rarely present as hyperosmolar hyperglycaemic state (HHS) (see ⊃ Chapter 12 on acute complications of T2D, pp. 208–212).

Early-onset type 2 diabetes

Diagnosis of T2D at an earlier age (under the age of 40 years) carries significant ↑ risks of mortality. There is an average of 11 years of life lost in those diagnosed at age of <20 years, and 7 years of life lost in those diagnosed at age between 20 and 39 years, compared with those without diabetes.[1] Early-onset T2D is a more aggressive diabetes phenotype than in older-onset presentations, resulting in a more rapid deterioration in glycaemic levels and a higher cardiometabolic risk factor profile.[2]

Young persons with T2D can face challenges in self-management that older individuals are less likely to experience such as being in education or of working age, higher diabetes distress, and possible obesity-related and diabetes-related stigma. Care needs to be individualized, taking into consideration these potentially ↑ challenges in care.

Signs and symptoms of type 2 diabetes

- Fatigue.
- Dry mouth/thirst.
- ↑ frequency of micturition, especially overnight.
- Recurrent mycotic infections.
- Recurrent general infections (e.g. skin, urine)
- Delayed wound healing.
- Periodontal disease.
- Deterioration in vision.
- Burning sensation/pain in feet.
- Unintentional weight loss.
- Erectile dysfunction.

References

1. Misra S, Gable D, Khunti K, *et al*. Developing services to support the delivery of care to people with early-onset type 2 diabetes. *Diabetic Medicine*. 2022;**39**:e14927.
2. Naveed S, Araz R, Stefan F, *et al*. Age at diagnosis of type 2 diabetes mellitus and associations with cardiovascular and mortality risks. *Circulation*. 2019;**139**(19):2228–37.

Principles of treatment of type 2 diabetes

Overall, the aim of care is to reduce the potential risk of micro- and macrovascular complications associated with T2D and to maintain quality of life.

- Look to the suitability to pursue a pathway for remission of T2D.
- Provide, or signpost to, T2D education and peer support to empower the person to make informed choices relating to their care.
- Screen for and, if required, provide or signpost to emotional and mental well-being support.
- Give access to holistic evidence-based lifestyle advice interventions to support management and reduce the risk of complications. This includes advice on activity, dietary, and circadian considerations.
- Look to set individualized, evidenced-based levels of attainment for blood glucose levels, blood pressure, lipid profiles, and renal function.
- Facilitate shared decision-making relating to lifestyle interventions and the use of medications in achieving desired levels and targets.
- Ensure ongoing review, as per evidence-based practice.

Management guidelines

Management guidelines support the principles of care as outlined above.

It is important that healthcare professionals (HCPs) are familiar with the most contemporaneous national, local, and global guidelines.

Current guidance from National Institute for Health and Care Excellence and is due to be updated at the time this book goes into print (NICE) is available at: ℘ https://www.nice.org.uk/guidance/ng28

The American Diabetes Association (ADA) and European Association for the Study of Diabetes (EASD) guidelines are available at: ℘ https://diabetesjournals.org/view-large/figure/5193638/dc25S009f3.tif

Both guidelines emphasize the importance of education, lifestyle, use of pharmacological therapies to support active cardiorenal protection (see ➲ Chapters 4, 11, and 12), use of anti-hyperglycaemic medication for individualized HbA1c attainment, and regular review.

Remission of type 2 diabetes

This is defined as HbA1c of below 48mmol/mol (6.5%) for at least 3 months apart and not having taken any glucose-lowering pharmacotherapy during this time.[1]

Even when T2D is in remission, it is important that a person still undergoes all diabetes health checks (see ➲ Chapters 9, 10, and 11) each year to include retinopathy screening to ensure that any complications that may have developed during the period of having diabetes are appropriately followed up and that T2D has not returned.

Remission of T2D is associated with weight loss changes, including that with metabolic surgery. Metabolic surgery appears to be effective for diabetes remission in people with T2D and a BMI ≥25kg/m², although the efficacy for both weight loss and diabetes remission appears to vary by surgical type.

The Diabetes Remission Clinical Trial (DiRECT)[2] was a structured primary care-led intensive weight management programme, which involved total diet replacement of 3452–3569kJ/day (825–853kcal/day) for 3–5 months, followed by stepped food reintroduction and structured support for long-term weight loss maintenance for persons diagnosed with T2D within the previous 6 years. It demonstrated greater remission than standard diabetes care, which varied with the degree of weight loss. At 2-year follow-up, those maintaining >10kg weight loss were more likely to still be in remission of T2D (65%). However, only 24% of participants in the intervention group maintained at least 10kg weight loss, highlighting both the potential and the challenges of long-term durability of weight loss.[2]

Diabetes education

Widespread research shows that structured diabetes education (SDE) in T2D improves knowledge, glycaemic levels, and psychological and clinical outcomes to include fewer hospital admissions and ↓ all-cause mortality.[3]

SDE may be delivered by local or national programmes as face-to-face groups or virtually. Both deliveries enable peer support, which again has evidence to support benefit.

Most providers offer culturally and disability-adapted programmes.

Technologies such as mobile apps, simulation tools, digital coaching, and digital self-management interventions can also be effective.

At diagnosis, and periodically throughout a person's journey in diabetes, it is important to look to signpost/refer to diabetes education, to enable shared decision-making and empowerment of the person with diabetes. It is desirable to extend this to families and/or carers.

References

1. Riddle MC, Cefalu WT, Evans PH, *et al*. Consensus report: definition and interpretation of remission in type 2 diabetes. *Diabetes Care*. 2021;**44**(10):2438–44.
2. Lean MEJ, Leslie WS, Barnes AC, *et al*. Durability of a primary care-led weight-management intervention for remission of type 2 diabetes: 2-year results of the DiRECT open-label, cluster-randomised trial. *The Lancet Diabetes & Endocrinology*. 2019;**7**(5):344–55.
3. Carey M, Khunti K, Davies M. Structured education in diabetes: a review of the evidence. *Diabetes & Primary Care*. 2012;**14**(3):154–62.

Lifestyle guidance

Dietary recommendations

Weight loss of 5–15% should be a primary target of management for many (but not all, depending on the BMI) people living with T2D.

There is no one specific dietary pattern that suits every person. It is important to individualize approaches based on factors such as acceptance of the person with diabetes, cultural preference, costs, access to cooking facilities/equipment, and understanding of the diet.

Studies have shown that Mediterranean and lower-carbohydrate diets have glycaemic benefits.[1]

(See ➲ Chapter 4 for further details relating to dietary advice in T2D.)

Smoking cessation advice and support as appropriate

- People who smoke with diabetes have ↑ CVD, premature death, microvascular complications, and more suboptimal glycaemic levels than non-smokers with diabetes.[2]
- T2D is more prevalent amongst people who smoke.

It is therefore important to ask people with T2D if they smoke, offer appropriate advice relating to risks to health, and signpost to local smoking cessation services if the person is in agreement for this.

Alcohol consumption review

To help keep health risks from alcohol at a low level, it is advised to keep within the national guidance of not regularly drinking >14 units of alcohol a week. The guidelines are the same for men and women, and recommend that if drinking up to 14 units a week, this is spread over at least 3 days.[3]

Review of any recreational drug use

Recreational drugs can affect glucose levels and the ability to self-manage diabetes care.

Physical activity

Physical activity is an integral part of the management of T2D.

Benefits

- Improved insulin sensitivity.
- Glycaemic benefits (especially if >45 exercise minutes undertaken postprandially).
- ↑ HDL levels.
- Facilitates weight loss.
- Improves cardiovascular health.
- Can have a positive impact on mood and help to relieve depression and stress.

Recommendations

- ≥150 minutes/week of moderate to vigorous aerobic activity. (Moderate activity is defined as any activity that leaves the individual slightly breathless, but still able to talk whilst undertaking the activity.)
- Or >75 minutes of vigorous-intensity activity spread over 3 days a week, with no more than 2 consecutive inactive days.

- Supplement aerobic activity with 2–3 sessions of resistance (i.e. using one's own body weight or working against a resistance), flexibility, and/or balance
- Interrupt periods of sitting every 30 minutes with light to vigorous activity.
- An ↑ of only 500 steps/day is associated with 2–9% ↓ risk of cardiovascular morbidity and all-cause mortality rates.[4]

Healthy sleeping patterns

Consistent, uninterrupted sleep confers benefit in T2D. However, sleep disorders, including sleep apnoea (which affects 24–70% of people with T2D), cause disturbances in the quantity, quality, and timing of sleep and are associated with an ↑ risk of obesity and disrupted glucose metabolism.

Adults should get at least 7 hours of sleep per night.

- Fewer than 7 hours of sleep per night regularly contributes to ↑ insulin resistance, feeling hungrier the next day, craving high-carbohydrate 'junk foods', lowered brain glucose use, and ↑ cortisol and sympathetic nervous system activity.
- Sleep deprivation (restriction to 5 hours' sleep for 7 nights) in healthy individuals results in a 20–65% ↓ in insulin sensitivity.[5]
- Energy intake is thought to be about 385kcal/day higher after partial sleep deprivation, with no change in energy expenditure or resting metabolic rate.
- Short sleep therefore makes it harder to lose weight—1-hour shorter sleep duration increases visceral adipose tissue mass by 0.11kg.
- Poor sleep is also associated with higher blood pressure, impairment of the immune system, and higher levels of depression and anxiety.

References

1. SchwingshacklL, Chaimani A, Hoffmann G, Schwedhelm C, Boeing H. A network meta-analysis on the comparative efficacy of different dietary approaches on glycaemic control in patients with type 2 diabetes mellitus. *European Journal of Epidemiology*. 2018;**33**:157–70.
2. Brown P. How to help people with diabetes stop smoking. *Diabetes & Primary Care*. 2021;**23**:13–14.
3. Department of Health and Social Care (2021). *Chapter 12: Alcohol*. Available at: 🖱 www.gov.uk/government/publications/delivering-better-oral-health-an-evidence-based-toolkit-for-prevention/chapter-12-alcohol
4. American Diabetes Association Professional Practice Committee. 5. Facilitating positive health behaviors and well-being to improve health outcomes: standards of care in diabetes—2024. *Diabetes Care*. 2024;**47**(Suppl 1):S77–110.
5. Reutrakul S, Punjabi NM, Van Cauter E. Impact of sleep and circadian disturbances on glucose metabolism and type 2 diabetes. In: Cowie CC, Casagrande SS, Menke A, *et al.* (editors). *Diabetes in America*, 3rd edition. Bethesda, MD: National Institute of Diabetes and Digestive and Kidney Diseases; 2018 Aug. Chapter 25. PMID: 33651564.

Further reading

The Diabetes and Nutrition Study Group (DNSG) of the European Association for the Study of Diabetes (EASD). Evidence-based European recommendations for the dietary management of diabetes. *Diabetologia*. 2023;**66**:965–85. 🖱 https://doi.org/10.1007/s00125-023-05894-8

Pharmacological management of hyperglycaemia

Hypoglycaemic agents have a variety of mechanisms of action to lower blood glucose levels. Each group of hypoglycaemic agents target specific organs/tissues to achieve this (see Fig. 2.2).

Metformin

• In most instances, first-line therapy in people with T2D.

Mode of action

• Reduces hepatic glucose production (gluconeogenesis).
• Reduces glucose absorption at gut level.
• Improves insulin sensitivity.
• Peripherally increases glucose uptake/utilization by skeletal muscles.

Potential benefits include

• Weight neutral, with potential for modest weight loss.
• Low risk of hypoglycaemia, unless used with insulin and/or a sulfonylurea.
• In UKPDS,[1] metformin showed a greater effect on any diabetes-related end point, including all-cause mortality and stroke.
• Low cost.
• World-established, with extensive clinical evidence.

Potential side effects include

• Gastrointestinal side effects (e.g. diarrhoea, abdominal cramping). Switching to a modified-release preparation might mitigate this if symptoms persist.
• Lactic acidosis is a rare, serious metabolic side effect that can occur because of metformin accumulation.
• Vitamin B12 deficiency and related worsening of neuropathy symptoms have been reported in some studies.[2]

Contraindications include

Metformin should be avoided for persons with:

• Renal complications (estimated glomerular filtration rate (eGFR) <30 and/or creatinine >130mmol/L)
• Hepatic failure
• Significant cardiac or respiratory failure.

Prescribing considerations include

• Starting dose should be low to facilitate tolerability and titrated in a timely manner as per the summary of product characteristics (SMPC) recommendations.
• Optimal effective dose is 2g/day.
• Metformin should not be used in people with eGFR <30mL/min/$1.73m^2$, and dose reduction to a total daily dose of 1g should be considered when the eGFR is <45mL/min/$1.73m^2$.
• Give sick day guidance to pause if any dehydrating/acute illness (see ➲ Chapter 17).
• Expected HbA1c reduction: 1–2% (11–22mmol/mol)[7].

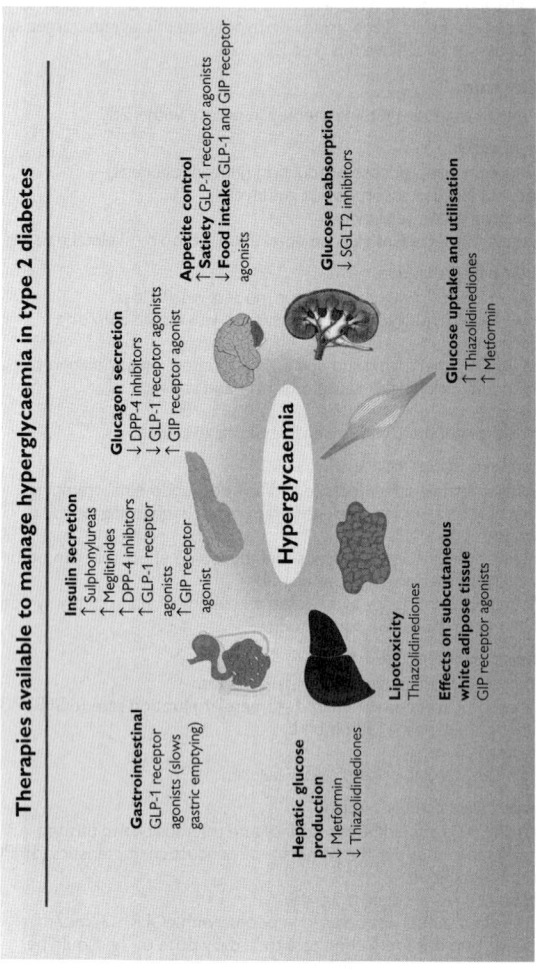

Fig. 2.2 Therapies available to manage hyperglycaemia in type 2 diabetes.

See British National Formulary (BNF)[3]/Electronic Medicines Compendium (EMC)[4]/SMPC for full prescribing information.

Sodium–glucose cotransporter 2 inhibitors

(canagliflozin, dapagliflozin, empagliflozin, ertugliflozin)

Originally used solely for glucose-lowering purposes, these medications now have evidence from various medication-specific cardiorenal outcome trials to show benefit beyond glycaemic improvement.

In respect of this, management guidelines now advocate for consideration/offer of a sodium–glucose cotransporter 2 (SGLT2) inhibitor, irrespective of glycaemic levels, to those at elevated risk of, or with established, atherosclerotic CVD (ASCVD), chronic kidney disease (CKD), and/or heart failure (HF) (see ➜ Chapter 10 on macrovascular complications and ➜ Chapter 11 on microvascular complications of diabetes).

It is important to consider the most efficacious SGLT2 inhibitor, based on the evidence base relating to the characteristics of the person for whom they are prescribed.

Mode of action
- Reduction of plasma glucose levels by enhancing urinary excretion of glucose.
- Glucose-lowering effect depends on renal function. There is lower glycaemic efficacy at lower eGFR.
- They work independently of β-cell function.

Potential benefits include
- Low risk of hypoglycaemia unless used with insulin and/or a sulfonylurea.
- Effective at all stages of T2D.
- Associated with:
  - Weight loss
  - Slight reduction in systolic blood pressure
  - Cardioprotection in established ASCVD*
  - Reduced rates of hospitalization in HF*
  - Renoprotection and cardiovascular protection in CKD.*

(* Not all SGLT2 inhibitors have demonstrated cardiorenal benefit. See ➜ Chapter 10 for which SGLT2 inhibitors have greatest evidence of benefit.)

Potential side effects include
- Genitourinary and mycotic infections.
- ↑ micturition.
- Postural hypotension.
- Rarely, euglycaemic diabetic ketoacidosis (DKA).

SGLT2 inhibitors should be avoided in the following instances:
- Situations where endogenous insulin production is compromised (e.g. type 1 diabetes, pancreatogenic diabetes, slowly evolving autoimmune-mediated diabetes)
- Previous DKA
- When renal function lies outside the indication for use (according to specific product licenses)

- Severe hepatic impairment[*]
- Acute illness/volume depletion
- Previous Fournier's gangrene (necrotizing fasciitis of the perineum)
- Recurrent fungal genital/urinary tract infection
- Pregnancy/breastfeeding
- Excessive alcohol intake
- Eating disorders
- Low-carbohydrate diet (e.g. ketogenic diet).

([*]Dapagliflozin 5mg can be used.)

Considerations when prescribing include
- Counsel on the risk of genitourinary infections and provide hygiene information.
- Advise to pause SGLT2 inhibitor treatment during acute and/or dehydrating illness and if required prior to surgical procedures.
- Advise to discuss with HCPs if considering starting on a very low-carbohydrate/ketogenic diet.
- Robust contraception for women of childbearing potential.
- Expected HbA1c reduction: 1–1.5% (11–17mmol/mol)[7].

See BNF[3]/EMC[4]/SMPC for full prescribing information.

Sulfonylureas

(gliclazide, glipizide, glimepiride, tolbutamide)
- This class of medication is well established, low cost, and has good glucose-lowering efficacy.
- May be used as 'rescue therapy' if having excluded type 1 diabetes, glucose levels are significantly raised, and there is symptomatic hyperglycaemia.

Mode of action
- Stimulate insulin secretion by binding to sulfonylurea receptors on the β-cell membrane.
- Require preserved β-cell function to achieve the above. May not be effective in later stages of T2D.

Side effects include
- Risk of hypoglycaemia.
- Modest potential weight gain.

Contraindications include
- Pregnancy and breastfeeding.
- Ketoacidosis.
- Severe renal and hepatic impairment.

Considerations when prescribing include
- Counsel on the risk of hypoglycaemia and provide related education, including on glucose monitoring (see ➔ Chapters 7 and 12 on the acute complications of diabetes).
- Advise on Driver and Vehicle Licensing Agency guidance (see ➔ Chapter 17).

- Ensure robust contraception for women of childbearing potential.
- Avoid in the frail/elderly due to the risk of hypoglycaemia (see ➜ Chapter 13).
- Expected HbA1c reduction: 1–2% (11–22mmol/mol)[7].

See BNF[3]/EMC[4]/SMPC for full prescribing information.

Incretin-based therapies

Dipeptidyl peptidase type 4 inhibitors
(alogliptin, linagliptin, sitagliptin, saxagliptin, vildagliptin)

Mode of action
- Inhibition of enzymatic inactivation of endogenous incretin hormones—protect native incretins from inactivation.
- ↑ insulin production in a glucose-dependent manner.
- ↓ glucagon secretion.

Potential benefits include
- Well tolerated.
- Weight neutral.
- Safety renal profile (can be used if eGFR <30—consult SMPC for doses).
- Low risk of hypoglycaemia.
- Cardiovascular safety (without benefit) demonstrated for all, except no data for vildagliptin.
- Can be used in frail, older persons.

Potential side effects include
- Angio-oedema/urticaria and other immune-mediated dermatological effects (e.g. bullous pemphigoid).
- Gastrointestinal side effects (abdominal pain, diarrhoea, reflux).

Contraindications include
- Ketoacidosis.
- Pregnancy/breastfeeding.

Considerations when prescribing include
- Dose adjustments required, depending on eGFR, except for linagliptin (refer to specific product licences).
- Not to be used concurrently with glucagon-like peptide 1 receptor agonist (GLP-1RA) therapy.
- Avoid saxagliptin and alogliptin in persons with HF.
- Expected reduction in HbA1c: 0.5–0.8% (6–9mmol/mol)[7].

See BNF[3]/EMC[4]/SMPC for full prescribing information.

Glucagon-like peptide 1 receptor agonists
(dulaglutide, exenatide, liraglutide, semaglutide)

What is the role of the incretin hormone glucagon-like peptide 1?
- ↑ insulin secretion and insulin sensitivity.
- ↑ β-cell mass and maintains β-cell function.

- ↑ glucose disposal.
- Delays gastric emptying.
- Reduces appetite by increasing satiety.

What are glucagon-like peptide 1 receptor agonists?

Chemical modification of glucagon-like peptide 1 (GLP-1) produces drugs that bind to the GLP-1 receptor, producing the same effects as the native protein. Current therapies all have a similar mechanism of action.

- GLP-1RA therapies are injectable, apart from oral semaglutide.
- They have different profiles, which affect the dosing frequency.

Potential benefits include

- Low risk of hypoglycaemia unless used with a sulfonylurea and/or insulin.
- Weight reduction.
- At the time of book going to print some therapies have demonstrated a reduction in major adverse cardiovascular events (MACE) (dulaglutide, liraglutide, and injectable semaglutide), and dulaglutide has demonstrated benefit in those at high risk of CVD (see ➔ Chapter 10 on macrovascular complications of diabetes).

Potential side effects include

- Gastrointestinal upset (e.g. dyspepsia, nausea, diarrhoea, constipation).

Contraindications include

- Pregnancy and breastfeeding.
- Pancreatitis.

Cautions include

- History of medullary thyroid cancer or multiple endocrine neoplasia type 2.
- Use with caution in pre-proliferative or proliferative retinopathy—non-significant ↑ in retinopathy with liraglutide vs placebo (hazard ratio, 1.15) in LEADER,[5] and a significant ↑ in retinopathy complications with injectable semaglutide when used with insulin (hazard ratio, 1.76) in SUSTAIN-6.[6]

Considerations for prescribing include

- Advise on mode of action and possible gastrointestinal side effects: explain that these are likely to reside with continued use.
- Give advice on how to minimize side effects (reduce portion sizes, avoid fatty and spicy foods).
- Explain the effect of earlier satiety.
- Advise on frequency of dosing and dose titration.
- Sick day guidance information (see ➔ Chapter 17).
- For injectable therapy, provide education on optimal injection technique (see ➔ Chapter 5).

- Ensure robust contraception for women of childbearing potential.
- Not recommended in diabetic gastroparesis.
- For suggested pathway for diabetic eye disease when starting GLP-1RA or combined glucose-dependent insulinotropic polypeptide and GLP-1RA, see guidance from the Primary Care Diabetes Society (PCDS) and Association of British Clinical Diabetologists. (See Fig. 2.3.)
- Expected HbA1c reduction: 0.8–1.5% (9–17mmol/mol).

See BNF[3]/EMC[4]/SMPC for full prescribing information.

Dual glucose-dependent insulinotropic polypeptide and glucagon-like peptide 1 receptor agonist
(tirzepatide)

Mode of action
Tirzepatide is the first in its class, being a single-molecule agonist of both the GLP-1 receptor and the receptor for glucose-dependent insulinotropic polypeptide (GIP). It is a weekly injectable therapy that is engineered to activate the GIP and GLP-1 receptors, which are key mediators of insulin secretion that are also expressed in the regions of the brain that regulate food intake.

Potential benefits include
- Low risk of hypoglycaemia unless used with a sulfonylurea and/or insulin.
- Weight loss.
- Cardiovascular benefit from improved lipid levels and blood pressure, and reduced visceral adiposity (further data on use in people with established CVD awaited at the time of writing).

Potential side effects can include:
- Nausea
- Vomiting
- Diarrhoea.

Considerations for prescribing include
- As per previous section for GLP1-RAs to include advice on minimizing potential gastrointestinal upset.
- Requirement for women living with obesity to switch to a non-oral method of contraception or adding a barrier method upon initiation for four weeks and for four weeks after any dose ↑.
- See pathway below regarding starting with diabetic eye disease (see Fig. 2.3).
- Expected HbA1c reduction: 1.9–2.6% (20–27mmol/mol).

See BNF[3]/EMC[4]/SMPC for full prescribing information.

**Suggested pathway for diabetic eye disease
when starting Rybelsus® or Mounjaro®**

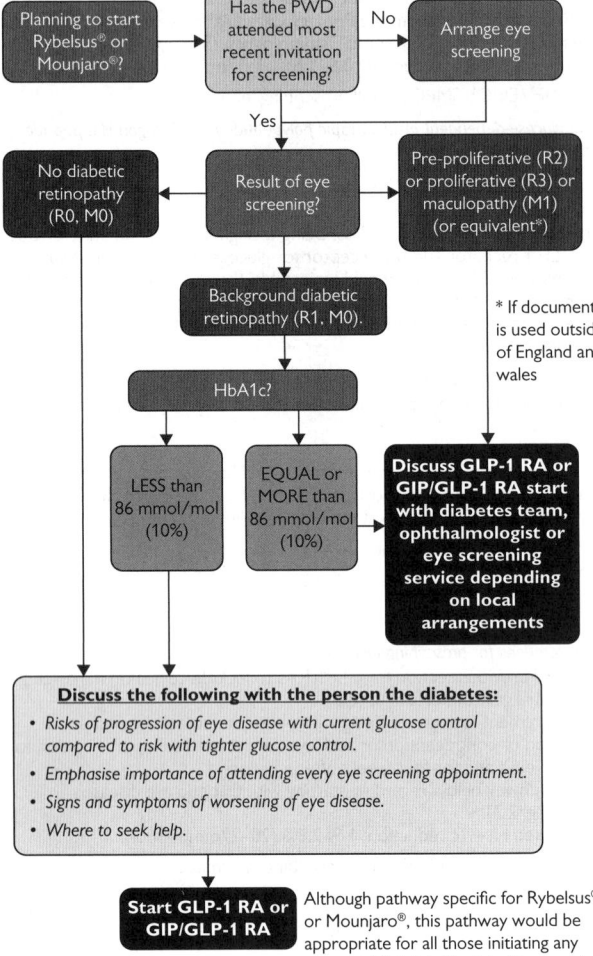

Fig. 2.3 Suggested Pathway for Diabetic Eye Disease.[7]

Thiazolidinediones (glitazones)

(pioglitazone)

Mode of action
- Insulin sensitizers that target adipocytes, muscle, and liver cells.
- Enhances insulin sensate genes.
- ↑ glucose uptake.
- ↑ adipocyte lipogenesis and ↓ circulating free fatty acids.

Potential benefits include
- Low risk of hypoglycaemia.
- High durability of glycaemic response.
- Beneficial effects on non-alcoholic fatty liver disease and non-alcoholic steatohepatitis.
- It can ↑ HDL and lower LDL and triglyceride levels.
- Can be used in renal impairment.

Potential side effects include
- Weight gain.
- Fluid retention leading to peripheral and macular oedema.
- ↑ risk of bone fractures.

Contraindications include
- HF or recent history of HF.
- Significant hepatic impairment (alanine aminotransferase >3 times the upper limit of normal).
- Pregnancy and breastfeeding.
- Avoid in persons with low bone density/osteoporosis, including post-menopausal women.
- Avoid if current, or history of, bladder cancer or unexplained haematuria.

Prescribing considerations include
- Caution in the frail/elderly (age-related ↑ risk of HF, fractures.
- Expected HbA1c reduction: 0.5–1.4% (5–15mmol/mol)[7].

  See BNF[3]/EMC[4]/SMPC for full prescribing information.

α-glucosidase inhibitors

(acarbose)
- Improve glycaemic levels by reducing postprandial glycaemic excursions and glycaemic variability. However, they are rarely used due to intolerable side effects, which include flatulence, abdominal pain, and diarrhoea.

Postprandial regulators

(repaglinide)
- Have a similar action to sulfonylureas (binding on different receptor sites in the β-cell). The onset of action tends to be faster, and they have a shorter duration of action.

- They are prescribed with meals, and doses can be adjusted according to the types of meals eaten.
- They are not commonly used.

See BNF[3]/EMC[4]/SMPC for full prescribing information.

References

1. King P, Peacock I, Donnelly R. The UK prospective diabetes study (UKPDS): clinical and thera-peutic implications for type 2 diabetes. *British Journal of Clinical Pharmacology*. 1999;**48**(5):643–8.
2. American Diabetes Association Professional Practice Committee. 5. Facilitating positive health behaviors and well-being to improve health outcomes: standards of care in diabetes—2024. *Diabetes Care*. 2024;**47**(Suppl 1):S77–110.
3. British National Formulary. Available at: ℘ https://bnf.nice.org.uk
4. Electronic Medicines Compendium. Available at: ℘ www.medicines.org.uk/emc#gref
5. Marso SP, Daniels GH, Brown-Frandsen K, *et al.* Liraglutide and cardiovascular outcomes in type 2 diabetes. *New England Journal of Medicine*. 2016;**375**:311–22. Available at: ℘ www.nejm.org/doi/full/10.1056/nejmoa1603827
6. Marso SP, Bain SC, Consoli A, *et al.* Semaglutide and cardiovascular outcomes in patients with type 2 diabetes. *New England Journal of Medicine*. 2016;**375**:1834–44. Available at: ℘ www.nejm.org/doi/full/10.1056/nejmoa1607141
7. Primary Care Diabetes Society, Association of British Clinical Diabetologists (2024). *Update March 2024: Glucagon-like-peptide 1 receptor agonist national shortage.* Available at: ℘ https://diabetesonthenet.com/wp-content/uploads/GLP-1-RA-Shortage-2024-ABCD-PCDS-FINALISED-170324.pdf

Insulin use in type 2 diabetes

The UKPDS demonstrated in 1998 that 58% of people with T2D required insulin within 14 years of diagnosis,[1] although it is important to consider that these findings were ahead of the use of more recent therapies such as SLGT2 inhibitors and GLP-1RAs. See ➲ Chapter 5 for full information on insulin use in diabetes.

Important considerations with all pharmacological therapies

- Medications only work when taken.
- Studies have shown that between 36% and 93% of people with T2D may struggle to take their medications as prescribed.[2]
- When initiating medications, it is important that education is given for the reason for the therapy and that decisions are shared.
- Consider individual person characteristics and health beliefs.
- Use of combination therapies, where available, may help to reduce pill burden.
- Ensure there is a scheduled review of treatment, with signposting of what to do if side effects are experienced.
- Consider that as a person's characteristics may change (e.g. with onset of frailty), medications may need to be deprescribed (see ➲ Chapter 13 on care in older persons).

References

1. Primary Care Diabetes Society, Association of British Clinical Diabetologists (2024). *Update March 2024: Glucagon-like-peptide 1 receptor agonist national shortage.* Available at: ℘ https://diabetesonthenet.com/wp-content/uploads/GLP-1-RA-Shortage-2024-ABCD-PCDS-FINALISED-170324.pdf

2. UK Prospective Diabetes Study (UKPDS) Group. Intensive blood-glucose control with sulphonylureas or insulin compared with conventional treatment and risk of complications in patients with type 2 diabetes (UKPDS 33). *The Lancet*. 1998;**352**:837–53. Available at: ℛ www.thelancet.com/journals/lancet/article/PIIS0140-6736(98)07019-6/fulltext

Further reading

Khunti N, Khunti N, Khunti K (2019). *Adherence to type 2 diabetes management*. Available at: ℛ www.bjd-abcd.com/index.php/bjd/article/view/391/671

Type 1 diabetes

Incidence and epidemiology

Type 1 diabetes (T1D) is one of the most frequently diagnosed chronic conditions in children, but the onset can be at any age. In adults, T1D can be misdiagnosed sometimes as type 2 diabetes (T2D) and accounts for ~5–10% of all cases of diabetes. The global prevalence is 5.9 per 10,000 people,[1] and the UK prevalence is currently 0.25%. There is also considerable geographical variation in incidence, with the highest number of cases reported in Finland and other Northern European nations and the lowest numbers reported in China and Venezuela.

The overall lifetime risk of developing T1D in a Caucasian population is currently 0.4%.[2] This risk increases to:

- 1–2% if the mother has T1DM
- 3–6% if the father has T1DM
- 5–6% if a sibling has T1DM
- Monozygotic twins have ~50% concordance rate by the age of 40 years.

The peak age for disease presentation is usually around puberty, with another peak between the age of 20 and 30 years.

References

1. Mobasseri M, Shirmohammadi M, Amiri T, Vahed N, Hosseini Fard H, Ghojazadeh M. Prevalence and incidence of type 1 diabetes in the world: a systematic review and meta-analysis. *Health Promotion Perspectives*. 2020;**10**:98–115.
2. Thanabalasingham G, Lumb A, Murphy H, *et al*. Diabetes. In: Owen K, Turner H, Wass J (editors). *Oxford Handbook of Endocrinology and Diabetes*, 4th edition. Oxford: Oxford University Press, 2021; pp. 837–980. Available at: ℞ https://doi.org/10.1093/med/9780198851899.003.0015

Aetiology

T1D is an autoimmune disease that leads to the destruction of insulin-producing pancreatic β-cells. The destruction can take place over months or years, eventually causing an absolute deficiency of insulin.

Although the exact aetiology is unknown, researchers believe that the human leucocyte antigen (HLA) genes of the major histocompatibility complex account for half of the heritability of T1D. The HLA class DR and DQ codes carry almost all of T1D susceptibility and >90% of people with T1D have at least one copy of these genes.

In those at risk, it is generally believed that viruses, dietary factors, and/or other stressors can trigger autoimmune β-cell destruction. Some studies have shown an ↑ risk of development of T1D related to infection with Coxsackie virus, enteroviruses, cytomegalovirus, rubella virus, influenza B, mumps virus, and more recently severe acute respiratory syndrome coronavirus 2 (SARS-CoV-2) (coronavirus disease 2019 (COVID-19)).[1]

Reference

1. Krischer JP, Liu X, Lernmark Å, *et al*.; TEDDY Study Group. Predictors of the initiation of islet autoimmunity and progression to multiple autoantibodies and clinical diabetes: the TEDDY Study. *Diabetes Care*. 2022;**45**(10):2271–81.

Presentation and diagnosis

Adults with new onset of T1D can present with the classical triad of poly-dipsia, polyuria, and weight loss, along with nausea, lassitude, and blurred vision.[1] The symptoms at the time of the first clinical presentation can usually be traced back several days to several weeks, even though β-cell destruc-tion may have started months or even years before this. If not evaluated and treated promptly, it can lead to diabetic ketoacidosis (DKA), which will require hospitalization to manage hyperglycaemia and electrolyte abnor-malities (see ➲ Chapter 12). Almost one-third of youth present with DKA.

Identifying whether an adult with newly diagnosed diabetes has T1D can be challenging at times, as some of the features, such as ketoacidosis, can also occur in ketosis-prone T2D.[1] Pancreatic cancer may present with hyperglycaemia and weight loss. Some adults with T1D maintain some in-sulin secretion for years after diabetes diagnosis and may not require insulin treatment at the time of diagnosis, which could lead to diagnostic uncer-tainty for some time. But accurate classification has other implications, including people obtaining access to newer technologies such as continuous glucose monitoring and the need for psychosocial support and access to other adjuvant therapies.

An initial diagnosis of T1D is made based on clinical grounds such as:[2]

• Ketoacidosis
• Rapid weight loss
• Body mass index below 25kg/m²*
• Personal and/or family history of autoimmune disease.

(* A higher BMI does not exclude T1D.)

People with T1D typically have one or more of the above.

Carry out further investigations such as serum C-peptide with a paired blood glucose and diabetes-specific autoimmune antibodies. Bear in mind that the false negative rate of diabetes-specific antibody tests is lowest at the time of diagnosis and C-peptide levels can be slightly elevated during the initial phase of T1D. If in any doubt whether a person has T1D, be safe and commence insulin.

(See Table 3.1)

Table 3.1 Differences between type 1 and type 2 diabetes

	Type 1 diabetes	Type 2 diabetes
Peak age of onset (years)	12	60
UK prevalence (%)	0.25	5–7 (10% of those aged >65 years)
Initial presentation	Polyuria, polydipsia, weight loss, ketoacidosis	Hyperglycaemic symptoms, often with complications of diabetes
Aetiology	Autoimmune β-cell destruction	Combination of insulin resistance, β-cell destruction, and β-cell dysfunction
Presence of β-cell antibodies	>90%	No
Insulin deficiency	Yes	Can develop after many years
Diabetic ketoacidosis	Common	Rare
Obesity	Uncommon	Common
Insulin resistance	Uncommon	Common
Treatment	Insulin from onset	Weight loss ± non-insulin hypoglycaemic agents ± insulin

(taken from Oxford Handbook of Endocrinology and Diabetes)

References

1. Holt RIG, DeVries JH, Hess-Fischl A, *et al*. The management of type 1 diabetes in adults. A consensus report by the American Diabetes Association (ADA) and the European Association for the Study of Diabetes (EASD). *Diabetes Care*. 2021;**44**:2589–625. Available at: 🔗 https://doi.org/10.2337/dci21-0043
2. National Institute for Health and Care Excellence (2022). *Type 1 diabetes in adults: diagnosis and management*. NICE guideline [NG17]. Available at: 🔗 www.nice.org.uk/guidance/ng17/chapter/Recommendations

Autoimmune antibodies

The presence of circulating pancreatic islet autoimmune antibodies suggests that the individual is at risk of, or has already developed, T1D. The antibodies responsible for causing T1D are:[1]

- Islet cell cytoplasmic antibodies (ICA)
- Insulin autoantibodies (IAA)
- Glutamic acid decarboxylase (GAD) isoform
- Insulinoma antigen 2 (IA-2)
- Zinc transporter isoform 8 (ZnT8).

These antibodies can be detected for a few years prior to diagnosis and frequently decline from the time of diagnosis. They can be absent in long-standing disease. GAD is the most common antibody detected in adults, with IAA being the more common one seen in children.

Autoimmune T1D is also associated with other autoimmune conditions such as thyroid disease, coeliac disease, Addison's disease, pernicious anaemia, and vitiligo. Appropriate screening must be done if any of these conditions are suspected.

Reference

1. Krischer JP, Liu X, Lernmark Å, et al.; TEDDY Study Group. Predictors of the initiation of islet autoimmunity and progression to multiple autoantibodies and clinical diabetes: the TEDDY Study. *Diabetes Care*. 2022;**45**(10):2271–81.

C-peptide

This is a marker of endogenous insulin and should always be measured with a paired glucose. The levels may vary, depending on insulin sensitivity.[1]

Generally, a random plasma C- peptide of <200pmol/L with a blood glucose level of >4mmol/L represents insulin deficiency and can be useful in confirming T1D (see Table 3.2 for C-peptide result interpretation).[1]

Table 3.2 C-peptide result interpretation

C-peptide (pmol/L)	Interpretation
<200	Severe insulin deficiency; confirms T1D; MODY unlikely
>600	Substantial endogenous insulin secretion. If duration >3 years, likely to be T2D or MODY
200–600	Likely T1D/insulin requiring. Also seen in long-standing T2D. Consider MODY if long-standing presumed T1D and antibodies negative

T1D, type 1 diabetes; MODY, maturity-onset diabetes of the young; T2D, type 2 diabetes.

Reference

1. Association of British Clinical Diabetologists (2020). *Standards of care for management of adults with type 1 diabetes 2020*. Available at: ℘ https://abcd.care/resource/standards-care-management-adults-type-1-diabetes-2020

Management

Insulin must be commenced as soon as the diagnosis is suspected/made. Urgent hospital admission is required for people with the following symptoms:
- Nausea/vomiting
- Increased respiratory rate
- Tachycardia
- Signs of dehydration
- Impaired conscious level

They will be assessed for DKA on hospital admission and a treatment pathway will be initiated according to hospital guidelines (see ➲ Chapter 12 for DKA management).

If none of the above symptoms are present, insulin can be initiated in the community or the person can be referred to the local diabetes specialist teams for this. All persons with newly diagnosed T1D must receive appropriate education from health care professionals specialized in diabetes. Multiple daily injections of basal (long-acting) and bolus (rapid-acting) insulin are the regimen of choice in most circumstances, commonly known as a multiple daily injection (MDI) regime (see ➲ Chapter 5). Insulin pump therapy can be considered as an option in the future if MDI therapy is considered impractical or inappropriate (see ➲ Chapter 6).

Education

Initial education should include:
- Insulin management
- Hypoglycaemia management (see ➲ Chapter 12)
- Sick day guidance
- Blood glucose and ketone monitoring (see ➲ Chapter 7)
- Basic diet management
- Key aspects of living with diabetes such as exercise, driving, work, alcohol, and pregnancy planning
- Link to peer support/support groups/online or written resources
- Follow-up plan with useful contact numbers.

The National Institute for Health and Care Excellence (NICE) recommends this should be followed by a validated, accredited, and quality-assured structured education course, which includes insulin dose adjustments according to carbohydrate intake, usually 6–12 months after diagnosis.[1] The DAFNE (Dose Adjustment for Normal Eating) programme was the first to establish the value of structured education, but other programmes, such as BERTIE and XPERT, are also delivered by many diabetes teams across the country.

Glucose monitoring

Guidance from NICE recommends the use of real-time continuous glucose monitoring (rtCGM) for adults and children with T1D.[1] But people should also be provided with a capillary blood glucose meter for testing during illness and times of rapidly changing glucose levels, and to check the accuracy of their real time continuous glucose monitoring (rt CGM) device (see ➲ Chapter 7, Continuous glucose monitoring, pp. 108–110).

Nutrition

All people with a new diagnosis of T1D should be referred to a specialist diabetes dietitian who will be able to provide individualized nutritional advice regarding healthy eating, the need for weight optimisation, and carbohydrate counting (see ➲ Chapter 4).

Physical activity and exercise

Advice should include insulin dose adjustment and dietary changes before and after exercise to reduce the risk of hypoglycaemia, the importance of regular glucose monitoring, and management of exercise-induced hyperglycaemia.

Sick day guidance and ketone monitoring

Stressful events, including illness, can affect glucose levels and increase the risk of DKA. More frequent glucose and ketone measurements are necessary to identify this. Individuals should be educated on sick day management at the time of diagnosis, and this should be discussed during follow-up consultations. Taking adequate amounts of fluids and carbohydrates, close monitoring of glucose and ketone levels, taking additional doses of insulin, and seeking urgent medical care are the main principles of sick day management. See Figs. 3.1 and 3.2 for examples of sick day guidance for persons on MDI regime and insulin pump therapy.[2]

Type 1 Diabetes: **Less guesswork.**
More freedom. Better health.

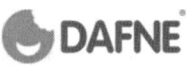

Sick day rules for standard DAFNE

SGLT2s may be prescribed by Consultants off licence to people with type 1 diabetes.
However, this flowchart is not suitable for people taking SGLT2 tablets (ending in –gliflozin),
please refer to the guidance provided by your local hospital.

Disclaimer

This guidance is developed for use by people with type 1 diabetes who have completed a 5-day
face to face DAFNE course[1] and understand the principles of accurate carbohydrate counting and
of insulin dose adjustment, so that their daily insulin doses are already balanced prior to following
this guidance.

The DAFNE programme assumes no responsibility or liability for any injury, loss, damage or
expense that may be caused by any action, or lack of action, that may be taken as a result of using
this guidance.

[1] delivered by appropriately trained and certified DAFNE educators.

Feel unwell?
Check blood glucose (BG) and ketones.

No significant ketones
(less than 1.5 mmol/L on blood check,
negative or trace on urine check)
BG within target or above target range
MINOR ILLNESS

Significant ketones present
(1.5 mmol/L or more on blood check,
more than a trace on urine check)
BG above target range
(usually above 13 mmol/L).
SEVERE ILLNESS

Sip sugar-free fluids (at least 100ml/hour).

Check BG and ketones every 4 to 6 hours.

Check BG and ketones every 2 hours.

Usual insulin: carbohydrate
ratio (QA:CP ratio) if eating.

If your BG is above target
range use QA corrections, even
if you are not eating (you may
find you need larger QA doses
to reduce BG).

If your BG is within target range
you may only need BI if you are
not eating.

Take your usual BI but you may
consider an increase in BI by 1
to 2 units if you continue to be
unwell for more than a day.

Calculate your 'typical' total daily dose (TDD).

Blood ketones
1.5–3.0 mmol/L
Urine ketones
small to moderate
+ or ++

Blood ketones
above 3.0 mmol/L
Urine ketones
large
+++ or ++++

Give 10% of TDD as
supplemental QA
insulin every 2 hours
plus usual QA:CP
ratio if eating, plus
usual BI.

Give 20% of TDD as
supplemental QA
insulin every 2 hours
plus usual QA:CP
ratio if eating, plus
usual BI.

If you vomit, are unable to keep fluids down, or are unable to control your blood
glucose or ketones you must go to hospital as an emergency.
You must never stop taking your BI.

Type 1 Diabetes: **Less guesswork.**
More freedom. Better health.

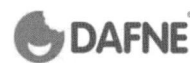

Sick day rules for Pump DAFNE

SGLT2s may be prescribed by Consultants off licence to people with type 1 diabetes.
However, this flowchart is not suitable for people taking SGLT2 tablets (ending in –gliflozin),
please refer to the guidance provided by your local hospital.

Disclaimer

This guidance is developed for use by people with type 1 diabetes who have completed a 5-day face to face DAFNE course[1] and understand the principles of accurate carbohydrate counting and of insulin dose adjustment, so that their daily insulin doses are already balanced prior to following this guidance.

The DAFNE programme assumes no responsibility or liability for any injury, loss, damage or expense that may be caused by any action, or lack of action, that may be taken as a result of using this guidance.

[1] delivered by appropriately trained and certified DAFNE educators.

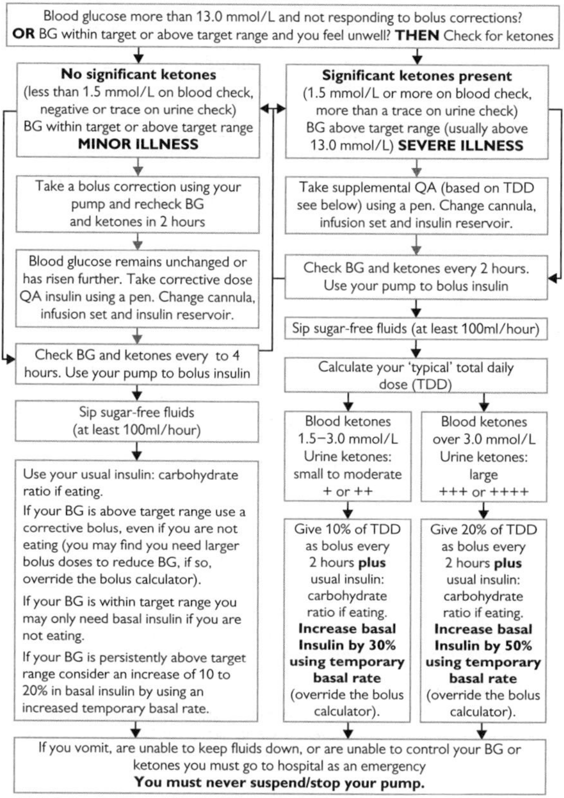

Blood glucose more than 13.0 mmol/L and not responding to bolus corrections?
OR BG within target or above target range and you feel unwell? **THEN** Check for ketones

No significant ketones (less than 1.5 mmol/L on blood check, negative or trace on urine check) BG within target or above target range **MINOR ILLNESS**	**Significant ketones present** (1.5 mmol/L or more on blood check, more than a trace on urine check) BG above target range (usually above 13.0 mmol/L) **SEVERE ILLNESS**

No significant ketones:

Take a bolus correction using your pump and recheck BG and ketones in 2 hours

Blood glucose remains unchanged or has risen further. Take corrective dose QA insulin using a pen. Change cannula, infusion set and insulin reservoir.

Check BG and ketones every to 4 hours. Use your pump to bolus insulin

Sip sugar-free fluids (at least 100ml/hour)

Use your usual insulin: carbohydrate ratio if eating.

If your BG is above target range use a corrective bolus, even if you are not eating (you may find you need larger bolus doses to reduce BG, if so, override the bolus calculator).

If your BG is within target range you may only need basal insulin if you are not eating.

If your BG is persistently above target range consider an increase of 10 to 20% in basal insulin by using an increased temporary basal rate.

Significant ketones:

Take supplemental QA (based on TDD see below) using a pen. Change cannula, infusion set and insulin reservoir.

Check BG and ketones every 2 hours. Use your pump to bolus insulin

Sip sugar-free fluids (at least 100ml/hour)

Calculate your 'typical' total daily dose (TDD)

Blood ketones 1.5–3.0 mmol/L Urine ketones: small to moderate + or ++	Blood ketones over 3.0 mmol/L Urine ketones: large +++ or ++++
Give 10% of TDD as bolus every 2 hours **plus** usual insulin: carbohydrate ratio if eating. **Increase basal Insulin by 30% using temporary basal rate** (override the bolus calculator).	Give 20% of TDD as bolus every 2 hours **plus** usual insulin: carbohydrate ratio if eating. **Increase basal Insulin by 50% using temporary basal rate** (override the bolus calculator).

If you vomit, are unable to keep fluids down, or are unable to control your BG or ketones you must go to hospital as an emergency
You must never suspend/stop your pump.

Fig. 3.1 and 3.2 "DAFNE sick day rules should be used as part of the DAFNE approach. In conjunction with DAFNE education the DAFNE Sick Day Rules are associated with ~80% reduction in episodes of DKA."

Ketones can be measured in the urine or blood, but the most accurate way of testing is by using a ketone meter that can check blood ketone levels. Urinary ketones can be inaccurate, especially in dilute samples and with dehydration and poor urine output.[3] NICE recommends the provision of a ketone meter and blood ketone strips for all adults with T1D to help with self-management of hyperglycaemia.

Blood ketones should be checked if blood glucose levels are above 15mmol/L (>13mmol/L if on insulin pump).

Table 3.3 contains useful reference levels for interpretation of blood and urine ketone tests.

Table 3.3 Useful reference levels for interpretation of blood and urine ketone tests

Blood ketone concentration (mmol/L)	Urine ketone (dipstick)	Interpretation
<0.6	Negative	Normal range
		Continue to check blood glucose levels and recheck ketones if glucose levels >15
0.6–1.5	Trace or +	Potential problem
		Follow sick day guidance and increase fluid intake
		Continue to check blood glucose levels and ketones 2-hourly. Seek medical advice if unwell
1.6–3.0	++	High risk of DKA
		Follow DAFNE sick day guidance and take extra doses of insulin
		Seek medical advice if unwell
>3.0	+++/++ ++	Likely DKA. Seek immediate medical help, especially if unable to keep fluids down

DKA, diabetic ketoacidosis.

References

1. National Institute for Health and Care Excellence (2022). *Type 1 diabetes in adults: diagnosis and management.* NICE guideline [NG17]. Available at: ℘ www.nice.org.uk/guidance/ng17/chapter/Recommendations
2. DAFNE (2020). *Sick day rules for standard DAFNE.* Available at: ℘ https://dafne.nhs.uk/wp-content/uploads/2020/03/HG-01-002-v3-Sick-day-rules-Standard-1.pdf
3. Diggle J. Ketones and diabetes. *Diabetes & Primary Care.* 2020;**22**:49–50.

Further reading

TREND-UK (2020). *Type 1 diabetes: what to do when you are ill* (patient information leaflet). Available at: ℘ https://trenddiabetes.online/wp-content/uploads/2020/03/A5_T1Illness_TREND_FINAL.pdf

Advanced therapies

Islet cell transplantation

Islets are separated from the donor pancreas and infused intraportally into the liver. Outcomes include improved glucose levels, and reduction in hypoglycaemic episodes and diabetes complications. The person will require immunosuppression. Individuals must fulfil specific criteria such as recurrent disabling hypoglycaemia despite optimal medical therapy, already on immunosuppression for renal transplant, or hypoglycaemia unawareness. According to the latest data, individuals are insulin-independent 1 year post-transplant, dropping to 50% at 4 years.

Pancreas transplantation

This is most commonly performed simultaneously with renal transplantation in people with T1D and renal failure. Ninety-five per cent of people are insulin-independent at 1 year, and 65–70% are insulin-independent at 5 years. These procedures must be carried out in centres with expertise in transplantation and diabetes management following multidisciplinary assessment.

Follow-up consultations

All people with T1D require ongoing care and support, appropriate to their age, from health care professionals experienced in the management of T1D. For most people, the follow-up consultation interval should be 6–12 months. An individual care plan should be agreed with the adult with T1D, and this should include:[1]

- Positive reinforcement and recognition of what the individual has already achieved
- Exploring any barriers to self-care management
- Identification of any diabetes-related distress (see ➲ Chapter 8)
- Review of individualized HbA1c target
- Review of blood glucose levels
- Insulin adjustment
- Assessment of hypoglycaemia awareness
- Review of lifestyle factors such as diet and exercise
- Review of technology use and the need for further updates
- Screening for any diabetes-related complications.

Reference

1. National Institute for Health and Care Excellence (2022). *Type 1 diabetes in adults: diagnosis and management.* NICE guideline [NG17]. Available at: ℞ www.nice.org.uk/guidance/ng17/chapter/Recommendations

Psychological support

The gold standard is that all individuals with T1D should have access to psychological care, but many areas do not have access to this. Despite the lack of resources, it is important that the clinician identifies psychological factors impacting diabetes self-management and appropriate referral is made to specialist psychological support (see ➔ Chapter 8).

Young adults and transition clinics

The transition from paediatric to adult diabetes service is a crucial time for all young people with diabetes and, if not carefully managed, can lead to adverse consequences such as not engaging with adult services. NICE recommends that the transition must be planned from age 13–14 years, with having annual meetings in respect of this. It also recommends that the practitioner from the adult service must meet young people in the paediatric setting before the transfer occurs.[1]

The paediatric Best Practice Tariff (BPT) is designed to raise standards of care for all children with diabetes up to the age of 19 years. Similar levels of care should be continued for several more years, even though most adult diabetes services struggle to provide similar standards of care. The requirements for a transition service are:

- Joint clinics with a paediatric and an adult diabetologist should be established
- A specialist young adult clinic for the 18- to 25-year age group should be held in a format and at a time that meet the needs of this age group
- Staff working in transition and young adult clinics should be trained in communication skills relevant to young people
- Psychological support should be available
- Attendance rates and outcomes should be audited.

Reference

1. National Institute for Health and Care Excellence (2023). *Transition from children's to adults' services*. Quality standard [QS140]. Available at: ⅋ www.nice.org.uk/guidance/qs140/chapter/Quality-statements

Further reading

NHS England (2016). *Diabetes transition service specification*. Available at: ⅋ www.england.nhs.uk/wp-content/uploads/2016/01/diabetes-transition-service-specification.pdf

Managing type 1 diabetes in older people

There is little evidence available on which to base guidance for management of T1D in older people.[1] Treatment should be individualized and must aim at reducing the risk of severe hypoglycaemia, assessment of vascular complications, assessment of frailty, and relaxation of targets. (see ➲ Chapter 13).

Reference

1. Association of British Clinical Diabetologists (2020). *Standards of care for management of adults with type 1 diabetes 2020*. Available at: ℘ https://abcd.care/resource/standards-care-managem ent-adults-type-1-diabetes-2020

Case study

Jenny is an 18-year-old university student, usually fit and healthy. She has been feeling extremely tired, thirsty, with a dry mouth and taking large amounts of fluids over the last few days. She consulted her General Practitioner (GP) as started feeling unwell with nausea and reduced oral intake. GP found glucose and ketones in the urine and advised to attend hospital.

On admission to the emergency department, a venous blood gas was completed, which showed: glucose 24mmol/L; pH 7.28; bicarbonate 16; and ketones 4.2mmol/L.

Question 1. How would you proceed to manage Jenny effectively?

- Jenny's admission symptoms are those of diabetes and the rapid onset of symptoms lead towards a potential diagnosis of T1D.
- The admission venous blood gas fulfils the criteria for DKA, which is a common presentation of newly diagnosed T1D.
- Initial management would include a fixed rate intravenous (IV) insulin infusion and fluids for DKA management. Long-acting insulin should be commenced and must be continued with an IV insulin infusion (see ⊇ Chapter 12).
- Urgent referral must be made to the inpatient diabetes team for education and support.
- Send blood samples for C-peptide, paired glucose, and autoimmune antibody testing to confirm the diagnosis of T1D.
- Once DKA has resolved, IV insulin can be safely converted to a regular subcutaneous insulin regime.
- The diabetes team should provide all basic education about diabetes, diet management, insulin injection technique, hypoglycaemia management, and glucose and ketone monitoring at home.
- Provide written diabetes information and signpost to appropriate online information and education.
- Identify an insulin regime which would be appropriate for Jenny to manage, according to her eating habits and lifestyle.
- Real-time CGM sensor to be provided, along with a blood glucose/ketone glucometer.
- Urgent review by an inpatient diabetes dietitian must be arranged, if available. If not, this can be arranged as an outpatient.
- Jenny must be given opportunities to safely practise insulin injections before discharge.
- Urgent referral to Jenny's local diabetes care team provider, and telephone follow-up must be arranged for initial support and for future care and management. Contact numbers to be provided to Jenny.

Dietary management of diabetes

Diet and diabetes

- In type 1 diabetes (T1D), dietary management can help to manage blood glucose levels and reduce the progression to potential T1D complications.
- In type 2 diabetes (T2D), it plays a key role in prevention, optimization, and possible remission. HbA1c reductions of up to 21mmol/mol have been reported as a result of diet/dietetic intervention.[1,2]
- Therefore, people living with any type of diabetes or at risk of developing T2D benefit from the support of a registered dietitian.
- There is no one-size-fits-all approach when it comes to diet, and evidence suggests it is the degree of adherence that predicts outcomes rather than the diet strategy.[3]
- It is therefore important that diet advice is acceptable, enjoyable, affordable, and 'adherable' if the aim is to achieve treatment goals and improve overall health.
- Structured diabetes education should also be made available to all people living with diabetes (see ➔ Chapters 2 and 3).
- Dietary management may differ slightly, depending on diabetes type, such as if the person is insulin-resistant or insulin-deficient.

For example:

Type 2 diabetes/generally insulin-resistant	Type 1 diabetes/insulin-deficient
• Calorie restriction to promote weight loss as appropriate and thus reduce insulin resistance • Reducing intake of processed foods and encouraging higher intakes of lower-kilocalorie, nutrient-dense foods—to promote satiety and weight loss • Moderate carbohydrate restriction to reduce postprandial glycaemia • Healthy eating to promote health and reduce risk factors such as raised lipids or blood pressure	• Healthy eating to promote good health and reduce risk factors such as raised lipids or blood pressure • Reducing intake of foods which cause rapid rises in blood glucose • Education on matching quick-acting insulin to carbohydrate-containing foods. Also known as 'carbohydrate counting' • If overweight/resistant to injected insulin, then also advice on calorie restriction to promote weight loss and reduce insulin resistance

There are a variety of diet strategies that are effective to achieve weight loss and improved blood glucose levels. For example, Dietary Approach to Stop Hypertension (DASH), vegetarian or vegan, the Nordic healthy diet, and moderate carbohydrate restriction. Overall, it is suggested that following a Mediterranean-style diet or an equivalent healthy eating pattern has the greatest evidence in terms of managing glucose levels and overall heart health.[4]

A Mediterranean diet focuses on:
- Reducing salt intake (<6g) a day
- Eating two portions of oily fish per week

- Eating more wholegrains, fruit and vegetables, fish, nuts, and legumes (pulses) (aim for >15g/1000kcal dietary fibre intake)
- Eating less red and processed meats
- Eating less refined carbohydrates and sugar-sweetened beverages
- Replacing saturated fats with unsaturated fats and limiting intake of trans fats (total fat should be <35% of total energy intake and saturated fats should be reduced to <10% of total energy intake)
- Enjoying alcohol, but limiting this to <14 units per week.

Diet and lifestyle tips

1. Do at least 150 minutes of moderate-intensity activity a week or 75 minutes of vigorous-intensity activity a week. Exercising ↑ energy expenditure, which can modify body composition favourably by ↓ fat mass and ↑ lean body mass. It can also reduce insulin resistance.
2. Aim for 2 litres of non-caffeinated fluid per day. It is important to stay well hydrated and it has been documented that many people will mistake thirst as hunger and can overeat if they are dehydrated.
3. Aim for 7–9 hours of sleep per night. Sleep loss creates a hormone imbalance in the body that promotes overeating and weight gain.[5]
4. Do not cut out wholefood groups or start strict diets without speaking to a health care professional. A balance of carbohydrates, fats, and proteins is necessary in our diets.
5. Very low-calorie diets have been shown to put some T2D into remission, but a medication review is important ahead of any such changes in dietary patterns, especially if taking medications associated with hypoglycaemia risk or a sodium–glucose cotransporter 2 (SGLT2) inhibitor.
6. Swap processed or refined foods for a more suitable alternative:

Swaps	Alternatives
Fruit juice/jams	Whole portion of fruit
White bread	Seeded, wholegrain, or rye bread
Mashed potato/potato waffle	New potatoes with skin or sweet potato
Cereals	Jumbo porridge oats
Ice cream	Plain Greek yoghurt
White/milk chocolate	Dark chocolate with >70% cocoa

Macronutrients

- Carbohydrates contain ~4kcal/g. They break down into glucose and can have a direct effect on blood glucose levels. The type and quantity of carbohydrate will affect blood glucose levels differently. People who monitor their blood glucose levels after meals or wear continuous blood glucose monitors may be able to see the effect different carbohydrate food and portions have on their blood glucose levels.

- Proteins contain ~4kcal/g. They break down into amino acids and do not have a direct effect on blood glucose.
- Fats contain ~9kcal/g. They break down into fatty acids and do not have a direct effect on blood glucose.
- Alcohol contains ~7kcal/g. Alcohol can cause blood glucose levels to fall.

References

1. Diabetes UK 2018 Nutrition Working Group (2018). *Evidence-based nutrition guidelines for the prevention and management of diabetes*. Available at: ℅ https://diabetes-resources-production.s3.eu-west-1.amazonaws.com/resources-s3/2018-03/1373_Nutrition%20guidelines_0.pdf
2. Dyson PA, Twenefour D, Breen C, *et al*. Diabetes UK evidence-based nutrition guidelines for the prevention and management of diabetes. *Diabetic Medicine*. 2018;**35**(5):541–7. doi: 10.1111/dme.13603.
3. Unwin D, Delon C, Unwin J, *et al*. What predicts drug-free type 2 diabetes remission? Insights from an 8-year general practice service evaluation of a lower carbohydrate diet with weight loss. *BMJ Nutrition, Prevention & Health*. 2023;**6**(1):46–55. doi: 10.1136/bmjnph-2022-000544.
4. Gibson AA, Sainsbury A. Strategies to improve adherence to dietary weight loss interventions in research and real-world settings. *Behavioral Sciences (Basel)*. 2017;**7**(3):44. doi: 10.3390/bs7030044.
5. Beccuti G, Pannain S. Sleep and obesity. *Current Opinion in Clinical Nutrition and Metabolic Care*. 2011;**14**(4):402–12. Available at: ℅ https://pubmed.ncbi.nlm.nih.gov/21659802/

Further reading

British Dietetic Association. Available at: ℅ www.bda.uk.com

Diabetes UK. Available at: ℅ www.diabetes.org.uk

Diabetes and Nutrition Study Group (DNSG) of the European Association for the Study of Diabetes (EASD). Evidence-based European recommendations for the dietary management of diabetes. *Diabetologia*. 2023;**66**(6):965–85.

Diabetes UK 2018 Nutrition Working Group. *Evidence-based nutrition guidelines for the prevention and management of diabetes*. Available at: ℅ https://diabetes-resources-production.s3.eu-west-1.amazonaws.com/resources-s3/2018-03/1373_Nutrition%20guidelines_0.pdf

Weight management and type 2 diabetes remission

- The most dominant predictor of T2D prevention is weight loss. Weight loss of 5–7% has been shown to reduce the relative risk of T2D by 50%.
- Evidence indicates high fat, high glycaemic index (GI), and low-fibre diets are associated with ↑ T2D risk.
- Diets that may protect against T2D include higher intakes of wholegrains, fruits, vegetables, yoghurts, cheese, coffee, and tea; also diets which are lower in red and processed meats, refined carbohydrate, and sugar-sweetened beverages.
- For people living with overweigt or obesity and T2D reducing energy intake to achieve weight loss should be the primary nutritional managment stragegy (see Fig, 4.1) It is important though, to note that sustained weight loss may need additional multiple support strategies to inlcude behaviour change and socio-econimic input.

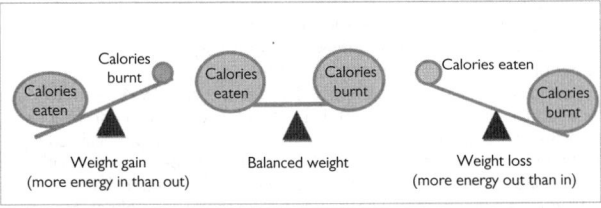

Fig. 4.1 Energy in vs energy out.

Weight loss of 5% or more improves:
- HbA1c
- Low-density lipoprotein (LDL) and high-density lipoprotein (HDL) cholesterol
- Triglycerides
- Blood pressure
- Insulin sensitivity.

T2D remission may be achieved if there is significant weight loss. It is thought that diabetes remission is due to ↑ β-cell function, associated with reducing fat stores in the pancreas and liver. Aiming for ~15kg weight loss as soon as possible after a diagnosis of T2D should be the goal for remission.

Very low-energy diets (VLEDs) have been shown to give a weight loss of up to 15kg, resulting in T2D remission. Total diet replacement (TDR) or meal replacement plans support the use of nutritionally complete liquid formula to provide 800–1200kcal/ day. VLEDs or TDR should only be used for a maximum of 12 weeks continuously or can be used intermittently. These diets should be followed with clinical and psychological support. Undertaking such diets without support may result in negative adverse outcomes, including severe hypoglycaemia and diabetic ketoacidosis (DKA).

Table 4.1 Glucose-lowering medications and their effect on weight

Medication	Effect on weight
Metformin	Neutral
DPP-4 inhibitors	Neutral
SGLT2 inhibitors	Reduction
GLP-1RAs	Reduction
Insulin	Gain
Pioglitazone	Gain
Sulfonylurea	Gain

DPP-4, dipeptidyl peptidase type 4; SGLT2, sodium–glucose cotransporter 2; GLP-1RA, glucagon-like peptide 1 receptor agonist.

Some diabetes medications are associated with weight loss/weight gain (see Table 4.1).

Bariatric surgery is recommended as a treatment option for adults living with T2D who have a BMI of 30kg/m^2 or more. T2D remission occurs in 30–62% of people following surgery. Bariatric surgery can also be offered to people living with T1D if clinically indicated.

Physical activity and/or exercise is associated with a 25–40% relative risk reduction in the development of T2D. Physical activity can also reduce insulin resistance and improve insulin sensitivity. However, physical activity in isolation is not an effective weight loss strategy for people living with diabetes unless they are exercising for 60 minutes or more per day.

Physical activity generally has a blood glucose-lowering effect. However, it may cause hyperglycaemia, hypoglycaemia, or a combination of both, especially in T1D.

Glycaemic management in type 1 diabetes

Carbohydrate can be found in a variety of foods (see Table 4.2). The quantity and quality of carbohydrate are the main nutritional consideration for people living with T1D in terms of desired glycaemic levels. People living with T1D should be supported to carbohydrate count and adjust insulin, depending on the quantity of carbohydrate eaten. Carbohydrate counting and insulin dose adjustment by using multiple daily injection (MDI) or continuous subcutaneous insulin infusion (CSII) allows for more freedom whilst maintaining desired glycaemic levels.

Table 4.2 Foods which do/do not contain carbohydrate

Carbohydrate-containing foods	
Starchy carbohydrates	Examples: pasta, rice, cereals, oats, grains, potatoes, breads, yams
Pulses and lentils (slow-releasing)	Examples: kidney beans, chickpeas, green and red lentils
Refined carbohydrates (quick-releasing)	Examples: sugar, honey, jams, boiled sweets, full sugar drinks, fruit juice
Fruit (fructose)	Examples: apple, pear, mangos, berries, bananas
Milk and some dairy (lactose)	Examples: cow milk, yoghurt
No or very low carbohydrate-containing foods	
Proteins	Examples: fish, chicken, eggs, tofu, lamb, pork
Fats	Examples: olive oil, nuts, cheese, avocado
Vegetables	Examples: onions, peppers, peas, broccoli, sugar snaps

For those on fixed doses of insulin, there should be an emphasis on meal timing and consistent carbohydrate portions per meals to achieve desired glycaemic levels.

Quick-releasing carbohydrate foods can cause postprandial blood glucose spikes and reduce time spent in range (see Fig. 4.2). Dietary and lifestyle variables, such as fat, protein, fibre, resistance starch, and activity, may help lower postprandial blood glucose levels after a meal. People with T1D should be offered education on how different carbohydrate types can have a different effect on postprandial blood glucose levels. Quick-releasing carbohydrate foods, such as fruit juice, jelly babies, glucose, and dextrose, should be used to raise blood glucose levels rapidly if levels drop below target (for hypoglycaemia management, see ➲ Chapter 12).

Additional nutrition recommendations may need to be considered for people with complications of diabetes:
- Diabetic neuropathy—advice on potassium, phosphate, salt, and energy intake as clinically required. Do not routinely restrict protein intake

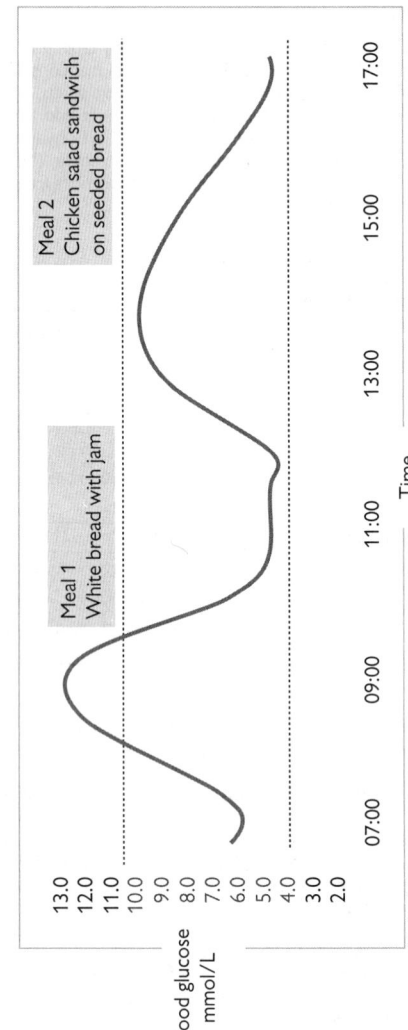

Fig. 4.2 Example of a blood glucose trace after two different meals.

- Lower limb amputations and ulcers—individual approach to minimize malnutrition and optimize glycaemic levels
- Diabetic gastroparesis—individualized care to meet requirements, manage symptoms, and optimize glycaemic levels. Consider low-fat/low-fibre meals, small frequent meals, complex carbohydrates, and energy-dense liquids in small volumes
- Nutrition support—aim to meet nutritional requirements and adjust diabetes treatment to optimize glycaemic levels. Diabetes-specific formula for enteral feeds can be recommended but are not routinely used in the UK
- Pregnancy—women living with diabetes should be offered dietetic support prior to conception and during pregnancy. Goals include achieving target HbA1c, weight loss preconceptionally if required, dietary advice, appropriate weight gain in pregnancy, and encouraging regular activity, including after meals, to lower postprandial blood glucose levels
- Coeliac disease—offer individualized advice to all people with coeliac disease and diabetes, and recommend a gluten-free diet
- Cystic fibrosis-related diabetes—individualized dietary and insulin education to optimize nutritional status and glycaemic levels.

Disordered eating

Eating disorders, such as anorexia, bulimia, and binge eating disorders, are up to 10 times more likely in people with T1D and T2D. Anyone can develop disordered eating; however, adolescents and young women are at greatest risk, with the prevalence estimated at 10–40%.

In T1D, reducing insulin doses or insulin omission used as an aid to lose weight is called diabulimia. Diabulimia can have serious consequences, including DKA and diabetes-related complications. Screening tools specific to diabetes have been developed (e.g. SEEDS, mSCOFF) to help identify disordered eating in T1D.

Specialist multidisciplinary team (MDT) support, including psychology care, should be sought for anyone identified as having, or at risk of, disordered eating.

Further reading

Juvenile Diabetes Research Foundation (2024). *Type 1 diabetes and disordered eating: Parliamentary Inquiry*. By Sir George Howarth MP and the Rt Hon. Theresa May MP. Available at: https://diabetes-resources-production.s3.eu-west-1.amazonaws.com/resources-s3/public/2024-01/TYPE1_A4_PAPER_JANUARY_2024_SCREEN.pdf

King's College Hospital NHS Foundation Trust. *Type 1 diabetes with disordered eating (T1DE)*. Available at: www.kch.nhs.uk/services/services-a-to-z/type-1-diabetes-with-disordered-eating-t1de/

Enteral feeding

Enteral feeding is commonly used in hospitals and can be essential to support adequate nutrition and recovery.

Managing glycaemic levels in people with diabetes receiving enteral feeding can be challenging and, if not managed appropriately, may slow patient recovery and potentially result in further complications.

- All people with diabetes receiving enteral feed should be reviewed by the diabetes specialist team, ideally in conjunction with the dietitian/nutrition team prior to commencing the feed to determine a suitable feed/treatment regimen.[1]
- Where possible, feeds should always be started at the prescribed time.
- Involve the diabetes specialist team immediately in the event of hypoglycaemia or recurrent hyperglycaemia.
- People with T1D or other insulin-deficient syndromes should never have their basal insulin omitted.
- Frequency of glucose testing whilst on the feed will depend on feed duration, type of diabetes, and diabetes treatment. More frequent monitoring may be required if the feed is unexpectedly switched off or glucose levels are below the recommended target range.
- There is a risk of hypoglycaemia if the feed is stopped or delayed for any unplanned reason. If the feed is interrupted and any feed-related insulin is still active, consideration of alternative ways of replacing carbohydrate until the feed can be restarted may be necessary (e.g. intravenous dextrose).
- Metformin liquid administered via an enteral feeding tube should be continued/commenced where appropriate. However, other oral hypoglycaemic agents should not be administered if the person is not eating a sufficient amount orally or is struggling to swallow.
- Crushing oral hypoglycaemic medications and administering via an enteral feeding tube is not advised and can result in unpredictable absorption and tube blockages.

Reference

1. Joint British Diabetes Societies for Inpatient Care (JBDS-IP) group (2024). *Glycaemic management during enteral feeding for people with diabetes in hospital: a guideline from the Joint British Diabetes Societies for Inpatient Care (JBDS-IP) group.* Available at: ℘ https://abcd.care/sites/default/files/resources/JBDS_05_Enteral_Feeding%20_Guideline_April_2024.pdf

Case study

Jenny, a 48-year-old female, went for a routine visit to the General Practitioner (GP) due to feeling more tired than usual. She has no other medical history and asked to get her bloods checked. Results over two tests showed she had a HbA1c of 52mmol/mol. Her GP explained the results and diagnosed her with T2D. Her GP asked some questions about her diet and lifestyle, and checked her weight and height to work out her BMI. Weight: 78kg; height: 1.6m; BMI: 30.5kg/m². Physical activity: works at a desk, swims for 60 minutes most Sundays. Diet: often skips breakfast or has a quick slice of white toast with butter; snacks mid morning with tea and biscuits or cakes, depending on what is in the office; lunch is usually a cheese sandwich and a packet of crisps; evening meals vary (e.g. pizza and chips, chicken, chips, and salad, sausage and mash). At weekends, drinks beer/cider ~8–10 pints over the weekend. And a takeaway on a Sunday.

Jenny was offered a place on the NHS Low-Kcal Plan 800kcal/day programme. However, she felt she would struggle to commit at this time and wanted some time to think about it. Her GP referred her to structured education and the dietitian, and planned a follow-up in 3 months' time to monitor and review.

After some education, Jenny agreed to some changes.
1. Aiming to ↑ swimming frequency to 2–3 times a week.
2. Aiming to have planned nutritious snacks (e.g. fruit, plain yoghurts) and limiting office biscuits/cakes to 1–2 times a week
3. Trying to add 1–2 veg at lunch and evening meal (e.g. swap cheese sandwich to egg salad sandwich)
4. Reducing alcohol intake to 14 units per week—also consider swapping alcohol choice. For example, swap 1 pint of beer/cider (~200kcal) for a spirit and sugar-free mixer (~70kcal)
5. Aiming to have lean protein at evening meal, such as grilled chicken, turkey sausages, white fish, eggs, and low-fat mince, and reducing higher-kcal options such as pizza, sausages, and fried meats.

On review, Jenny's weight had reduced by 8kg (10%) in 3 months. Her BMI was now 27kg/m², and her repeated HbA1c had reduced to 46mmol/mol. Further HbA1c 3 months later was 45mmol/mol. Jenny's T2D was now in remission but remained in the non-diabetic hyperglycaemic range. Her GP offered a 6-month review and encouraged further weight loss. Jenny's GP referred her to a physical activity referral scheme, as she was feeling more confident to explore other forms of exercise.

Chapter 5

Insulin use in diabetes

Introduction

Prior to the discovery and development of insulin, people with type 1 diabetes (T1D) often died within a few weeks or months of diagnosis. The only treatment available at the time was complete removal of carbohydrate from the diet. The discovery of insulin in 1920 is one of the greatest medical breakthroughs in history, saving millions of lives around the world.

- T1D requires immediate and lifelong insulin treatment.
- In type 2 diabetes (T2D), there is typically a gradual decline in insulin production that often coexists with insulin resistance. Many people with T2D eventually require insulin therapy. Although the increasing number of non-insulin-based therapies can delay the progression to insulin in T2D.
- With the rising prevalence of diabetes and an increasing life expectancy, the absolute number of individuals using insulin is rising.

Up until the early 1980s, animal insulin (mostly pork and bovine) was used, but supply problems and allergic reactions for many led to the development of 'human insulins', the first of which was Humulin® in 1982.

Genetically engineered insulins, which more closely matched endogenous insulin, followed in the mid-nineties, initially rapid-acting insulins and, by the millennium, long-acting analogue insulin.

Currently, *there are over 30 different insulin preparations*, including higher-concentration insulins and biosimilar insulins.

- Despite similar-sounding names, time action profiles and recommended timing of administration may be very different. Therefore, great attention to detail is required when insulin is prescribed and administered.
- Insulin is recognized as a high-risk medication, with the potential to cause severe harm or even death. Incorrect dosing, imprecise or illegible prescription, or administration error can all cause patient harm or near-miss injury.

It is imperative that insulin therapy is only ever initiated and managed by health care professionals with relevant expertise and training.

All health care workers who handle, prescribe, or administer insulin should receive regular training and demonstrate competence.

When is insulin needed?

- A person with T1D is dependent upon insulin to survive, and insulin will be required immediately (except for slowly evolving, immune-related diabetes when it may be delayed (see ➲ Chapter 1).
- Insulin deficiency tends to occur gradually in people with T2D. Therefore, the optimal time to begin insulin therapy is not clearly defined or easily recognized. However, insulin should be considered in those with T2D:
  - When blood glucose levels are inadequately controlled despite being on maximum tolerated non-insulin-based antidiabetes therapy (including, where appropriate, glucagon-like peptide 1 receptor agonists), or
  - Where non-insulin-based glucose lowering drugs are contraindicated or not tolerated.

Importantly, insulin is effective where other agents are not and should be considered as part of any combination regimen, but especially where glucose levels are ≥16.7mmol/L or HbA1c is ≥86mmol/mol or when a person is experiencing symptoms of hyperglycaemia, including polyuria or polydipsia.

Insulin may be used as *rescue therapy* at any phase of treatment in adults with T2D who are symptomatically hyperglycaemic, including at diagnosis or early in treatment, and its ongoing requirement should be reassessed later.

The decision to initiate insulin in those with T2D will usually be driven by the following:[1]

- Deteriorating glycaemic levels
- Symptomatic hyperglycaemia
- Persistently elevated HbA1c despite optimal intensification of non-insulin blood glucose-lowering drugs or intolerance to these drugs
- Personal preference
- Pregnancy or planning pregnancy
- During acute illness
- Treatment with steroid therapy.

In practice, there is often a delay in intensifying T2D treatment, especially progression to insulin, with delays of over 7 years despite very high baseline HbA1c levels.[2,3]

Reasons why clinicians may be reluctant to start insulin therapy in T2D include:

- Underestimation of the need for treatment intensification
- Collusion with individuals who are reluctant to start insulin
- Confusion over guidelines
- Lack of knowledge or confidence around prescribing insulin
- Practical challenges, including dosing and injection technique
- Time constraints
- Lack of resources, including workforce with required skills and competency
- Concerns over adverse effects (particularly hypoglycaemia and weight gain).

Individuals living with T2D may also have barriers to starting insulin, including:

- Denial of the condition (absence of symptoms—feeling fine)
- Belief the condition is not serious
- Concerns over the inconvenience and negative impact on quality of life
- Worry about side effects (especially the fear of hypoglycaemia and weight gain)
- Poor understanding of the benefits of insulin
- Influence of external factors (e.g. internet, negative or inaccurate media coverage, family and friends' experiences of insulin therapy)
- Worry over employment restrictions and/or driving
- Anxiety about injecting and fear of needles
- Social inconvenience and/or embarrassment of having to inject insulin
- Incorrect perception that insulin is a punishment for 'suboptimal diabetes levels'.

A useful strategy is to discuss the possibility of insulin therapy in T2D early, as this gives a person time to get used to the idea and an opportunity to discuss any reservations or fears they may have. The following open questions are useful prompts for these conversations:[4]

- What is your greatest concern about starting insulin?
- What are the obstacles to/would stop you from using insulin?
- How confident are you about using insulin?
- What information/support do you need to try an injectable therapy?

Many people can be anxious about self-injecting and worry about needles, so it can help to show the modern pen devices and needles, and even give an opportunity to perform a 'dummy injection'. Importantly, health care professionals should NEVER use insulin therapy as a threat in an attempt to improve a person's glycaemic levels.

References

1. National Institute for Health and Care Excellence (2016). *Insulin therapy in type 2 diabetes*. NICE Clinical Knowledge Summaries. Available at: 🔗 cks.nice.org.uk/insulin-therapy-in-type-2-diabetes
2. Calvert MJ, McManus RJ, Freemantle N. Management of type 2 diabetes with multiple oral hypoglycaemic agents or insulin in primary care: retrospective cohort study. *British Journal of General Practice*. 2007;**57**:455–60.
3. Khunti K, Wolden ML, Thorsted BL, Andersan M, Davies MJ. Clinical inertia in people with type 2 diabetes: a retrospective cohort study of more than 80,000 people. *Diabetes Care*. 2013;**36**:3411–17.
4. Kruger DF, LaRue S, Estepa P. Recognition of and steps to mitigate anxiety and fear of pain in injectable diabetes treatment. *Diabetes, Metabolic Syndrome and Obesity*. 2015;**8**:49–56.

Different insulin types and regimens

For a complete list of insulins and delivery devices and up-to-date pre-scribing information, refer to British National Formulary (available at: ✏ www.bnf.org). Refer to each insulin's specific summary of product charac-teristics (SMPC) (available at: ✏ www.medicines.org.uk).

There are five broad categories of insulin defined by the preparation's 'time–action profile', which includes the onset of action, peak activity, and duration of action.

Mealtime or 'bolus' insulin is either short- or rapid-acting insulin, usually given in combination with one or two separate daily injections of inter-mediate- or long-acting insulin.

An approximate guide to onset of action, peak activity, and duration of action for different types of insulin is shown in Table 5.1 and Fig. 5.1. *However, these vary with individual products and it is important to refer to the manufacturer's guidance for individual products.*

Higher-concentration insulin

The insulin preparation most commonly used in the UK is 100 units/mL, which delivers 100 units of insulin in 1mL. However, insulins are available in the UK that deliver 200 units of insulin in 1mL and 300 units of insulin in 1mL. Higher-concentration insulin is becoming more common and has the advantage of containing the same amount of insulin in less volume. This is particularly useful for individuals on larger doses of insulin.

There are currently three types of insulin available as a 200 units/mL concentration:
- Humalog® 200 units/mL (insulin lispro) is a rapid-acting mealtime insulin, available only in the prefilled KwikPen® device.
- Tresiba® 200 units/mL (insulin degludec) is a long-acting insulin, available only in the prefilled FlexTouch® device. This device can be used to dial up to 160 units in 2-unit increments.
- Lyumjev® 200 units/mL (insulin lispro) is an ultrarapid-acting mealtime insulin, available only in the prefilled KwikPen® device.

Currently, there is one insulin available as a 300 units/mL concentration:
- Toujeo® 300 units/mL (insulin glargine) is a long-acting basal insulin, with a flatter profile than Lantus® 100 units/mL (insulin glargine). It should be taken once daily and has a duration of action of 36 hours. It is not bioequivalent to Lantus® and therefore is not interchangeable.

Humulin-R® U500 (as a 500 units/mL concentration of soluble insulin, nor-mally injected three times daily before meals) is available from the United States but can only be prescribed by a consultant on a named-person basis (this insulin is not licensed in the UK).

To reduce errors, higher-concentration insulins are only available in prefilled pen devices. The dial on the pen will give the correct dose, and the dose required (in units) should not be adjusted for different concentrations of insulin.

Insulin should *NEVER* be withdrawn from a cartridge or insulin pen by using a syringe and needle.

Table 5.1 Insulin types and available medicinal forms in the UK

	Insulin Type & Available Medicinal Forms in the UK		**Diabetes Specialist** Nurse Forum UK
Insulin action	Insulin brand name & manufacturer	Delivery device	*compatible re-usable cartridge pen device
Ultra-Rapid	**Fiasp** (aspart) Manufacturer: Novo Nordisk	FlexTouch Pen 3ml Penfill cartridge* 10ml vial	NovoPen 6 NovoPen Echo Plus
	Lyumjev 100 units/ ml (lispro) Manufacturer: Eli Lilly	KwikPen Junior KwikPen 3ml cartridge* 10ml vial	HumaPen Savvio
	Lyumjev 200 units/ ml (lispro) Manufacturer: Eli Lilly	KwikPen	N/A
Rapid	**Admelog** (lispro) Manufacturer: Sanofi	SoloStar Pen 3ml cartridge* 10ml vial	All Star PRO Junior STAR
	Apidra (glulisine) Manufacturer: Sanofi	SoloStar Pen 3ml cartridge* 10ml vial	All Star PRO Junior STAR
	Humalog 100 units/ ml (lispro) Manufacturer: Eli Lilly	KwikPen Junior KwikPen 3ml cartridge* 10ml vial	HumaPen Savvio
	Humalog 200 units/ ml (lispro) Manufacturer: Eli Lilly	KwikPen	N/A
	NovoRapid (aspart) Manufacturer: Novo Nordisk	FlexPen FlexTouch Pen 3ml Penfill cartridge* 10ml vial 1.6ml PumpCart	NovoPen 6 NovoPen Echo Plus
	Trurapi (aspart) Manufacturer: Sanofi	SoloStar Pen 3ml cartridge* 10ml vial	All Star PRO Junior STAR
Short	**Actrapid** (insulin soluble human) Manufacturer: Novo Nordisk	10ml vial	N/A

Table 5.1 (*Contd.*)

Insulin action	Insulin brand name & manufacturer	Delivery device	*compatible re-usable cartridge pen device
	Humulin S (soluble human) Manufacturer: Eli Lilly	3ml cartridge* 10ml vial	HumaPen Savvio
	Hypurin Porcine Neutral (soluble porcine) Manufacturer: Wockhardt	3ml cartridge* 10ml vial	Autopen Classic
Inter-mediate	**Humulin I** (isophane human) Manufacturer: Eli Lilly	KwikPen 3ml cartridge* 10ml vial	HumaPen Savvio
	Insulatard (isophane human) Manufacturer: Novo Nordisk	3ml Penfill cartridge* 10ml vial	NovoPen 6 NovoPen Echo Plus
	Hypurin Porcine Isophane (isophane porcine) Manufacturer: Wockhardt	3ml cartridges 10ml vial	Autopen Classic
Basal	**Abasaglar** (glargine) Manufacturer: Eli Lilly	KwikPen 3ml cartridge*	HumaPen Savvio
	Lantus (glargine) Manufacturer: Sanofi	SoloStar Pen 3ml cartridge* 10ml vial	All Star PRO Junior STAR
	Levemir (detemir) Manufacturer: Novo Nordisk	FlexPen 3ml Penfill cartridge*	NovoPen 6 NovoPen Echo Plus
	Toujeo 300 units/ml (insulin glargine 300 units/ml) Manufacturer: Sanofi	SoloStar DoubleStar	N/A
	Tresiba 100 units/ml (degludec) Manufacturer: Novo Nordisk	FlexTouch Pen 3ml Penfill cartridge*	NovoPen 6 NovoPen Echo Plus
	Tresiba 200 units/ml (degludec 200 units/ml) Manufacturer: Novo Nordisk	FlexTouch Pen	N/A

(Continued)

Table 5.1 (Contd.)

Insulin action	Insulin brand name & manufacturer	Delivery device	*compatible re-usable cartridge pen device
	Semglee (glargine) Manufacturer: Viatris	Pre-filed Pen	N/A
Pre-mixed Analogues	**NovoMix 30** (aspart protamine) Manufacturer: Novo Nordisk	FlexPen 3ml cartridge*	NovoPen 6 NovoPen Echo Plus
	Humalog Mix 25 (lispro protamine) Manufacturer: Eli Lilly	KwikPen 3ml cartridge* 10ml vial	HumaPen Savvio
	Humalog Mix 50 (lispro protamine) Manufacturer: Eli Lilly	KwikPen 3ml cartridge*	HumaPen Savvio
Pre-mixed Human	**Humulin M3** (soluble/isophane human) Manufacturer: Eli Lilly	KwikPen 3ml cartridge* 10ml vial	HumaPen Savvio
	Hypurine Procine 30/70 Mix (soluble/isophane procine) Manufacturer: Wockhardt	3ml cartridge* 10ml vial	AutoPen Classic

*Re-Usable cartridge pens can only be used with company specific insulin 3ml cartridges

With kind permission from DSN Forum to reproduce – ℛ https://www.diabetesspecialistnurse forumuk.co.uk/charts

*At the time of publication, insulin levemir (in all device formats) is expected to be discontinued and novo-rapid insulin will no longer be available in the flex touch pen device. Insulin hypurin is also unlikely to be available.

Biosimilar insulin

A biosimilar product is a biological copy that is not identical, but demonstrates similarity, to the original product in terms of quality, efficacy, and safety.

The following biosimilar insulins are currently available in the UK:
- Abasaglar® (insulin glargine injection—recombinant DNA (rDNA) origin, 100 units/mL)
- Semglee® (insulin glargine injection—rDNA origin, 100 units/mL)
- Admelog® (insulin lispro injection—rDNA origin, 100 units/mL)
- Trurapi® (insulin aspart injection—rDNA origin, 100 units/mL).

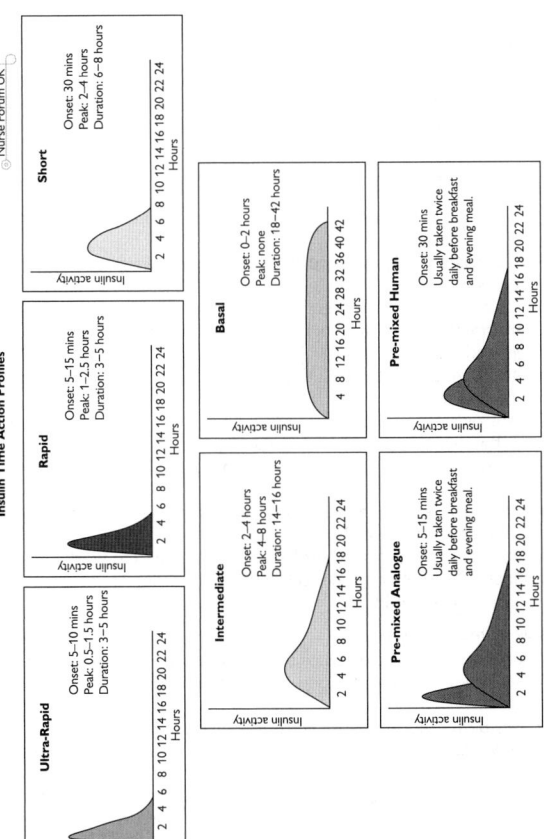

Fig. 5.1 Insulin time-action profiles.

With kind permission from DSN Forum to reproduce – ℗ https://www.diabetesspecialistnurseforumuk.co.uk/charts

Insulin regimen options

Type 1 diabetes: basal bolus or continuous subcutaneous insulin infusion*

(* A continuous insulin regimen—individuals on this regimen should be managed by a specialist team; see ➲ Chapter 6)

Type 2 Diabetes

Once- or twice-daily basal insulin

Commonly used as first-line insulin treatment for people with T2D, with or without other non-insulin diabetes medications.

- Simple and easy to teach.
- Initially requires only one injection per day, which may be beneficial in individuals who are reluctant to start insulin or are fearful about injections or those requiring someone else to administer (e.g. district nurse).
- May be associated with less hypoglycaemia and less weight gain than other regimens.
- If given at bedtime, this will predominantly target fasting hyperglycaemia and therefore is most useful when blood glucose levels are high overnight and in the morning.
- When given once daily, the best time to administer it is in the evening or before bedtime.
- If using steroids, a morning dose is more effective as glucose levels tend to rise in the morning and fall later in the day.
- Less effective in addressing the rise in blood glucose level that occurs after meals.
- Some individuals may not achieve optimal glucose levels with once-daily dosing and require twice-daily or more dosing.
- Basal analogues have a 'flatter' profile and are designed to work throughout a 24- to 42-hour period (duration of action varies—refer to individual product's SMPC).

Twice-daily premixed insulin

These insulins are usually given twice daily, before breakfast and before the evening meal; they may also be used once daily or three times daily (with each meal).

- Potentially better blood glucose levels following meals.
- May be preferable to basal insulin alone in those with particularly high HbA1c (>75mmol/mol).
- Can be initiated as one injection per day to familiarize the individual, with additional injections added later to optimize glucose levels.
- Less flexible than basal bolus regimens because short- and longer-acting insulin components cannot be adjusted independently.
- Lunchtime glucose level rise may not be covered with twice-daily dosing.
- May be more difficult to teach dose adjustment and titration, as individuals must adjust the insulin injection that precedes the high blood

glucose reading (e.g. where there is a pattern of high readings before the evening meal, then the morning insulin dose should be adjusted).
- The need to inject 20–30 minutes before a meal may be inconvenient for some individuals.
- There may be a need for snacks between meals to avoid hypoglycaemia.
- Better suited for people with regular lifestyles, who eat similar amounts of carbohydrate at similar times each day.
- Premixed analogue insulins may be given 15 minutes before a meal, which may be more convenient, and the shorter duration of action of the mealtime insulin component may reduce the need for snacks to avoid hypoglycaemia.
- Individuals on a premixed insulin regimen should be monitored for the need for a further injection of short-acting insulin at lunchtime or for a change to basal bolus if blood glucose levels remain suboptimal.

Basal bolus/multiple-dose insulin regimens
These require the individual to take a once- or twice-daily intermediate- or long-acting insulin to provide background insulin and then rapid- or short-acting insulin to cover mealtimes.
- This regimen produces an insulin profile that is closest to the body's natural insulin production.
- The mealtime and basal insulin may be adjusted independently, thus offering greater flexibility over the type of food and when it can be eaten.
- Multiple insulin injections require commitment and motivation.
- More frequent glucose monitoring and dose adjustment are needed.
- May be associated with more hypoglycaemia and greater weight gain than other regimens.
- Requires a good understanding of the impact of food choices, including portion sizes and carbohydrate awareness.
- Sulfonylureas should be stopped when mealtime or premixed insulin is added, and doses may need to be reduced when basal insulin is added.

Insulin delivery devices

Insulin can be administered by using insulin syringes, cartridges for reusable insulin pens, prefilled disposable insulin pens, infusion sets, and insulin pumps (see ➲ Chapter 6 for infusion sets and insulin pumps).

- Insulin syringes are specially designed for administering insulin. U100 insulin syringes hold up to 1mL or 100 units of insulin. There are also other types of insulin syringes available such as 0.5mL (50 units) and 0.3mL (30 units). The correct syringe for the dose given by the graduation on individual syringes allows for safe measurement of the dose. The size of the syringe used should be aligned with the individual amount of insulin to be injected (e.g. very small doses will need only a 0.3mL syringe).
- The insulin is drawn up into the syringe from a vial.
- These syringes have a fixed needle already fitted (some of these syringes will have a safety needle included)—due to the length of the needles, a lifted skinfold technique should be used.
- Following injection, they should be disposed of by using a sharps container. The needle should never be resheathed because of the risk of needle-stick injury.
- More commonly, in practice, insulin is administered from a cartridge pen or prefilled pen. Insulin pens can be used to give up to 50, 60, 80, or 160 units in 0.5-, 1-, or 2-unit increments (see Tables 5.2 and 5.3).
- Cartridges, for use in non-disposable pens, are available in packs of five and contain 100 units per mL, giving a total 300 units in 3mL. Each cartridge is clearly marked, so that the user can tell how much insulin is left in each.
- Most disposable prefilled pens also contain 300 units in 3mL, apart from Tresiba® 200 units/mL FlexTouch® and the Humalog® 200 units/mL KwikPen®, both of which hold 600 units, the Toujeo® 300 units/mL SoloStar® device which holds 450 units, and the DoubleStar® device which holds 900 units. The entire pen device should be discarded when the insulin is used up.
- Single-use disposable pen needles must be prescribed separately. These are available in a variety of sizes (gauge and length).
- Insulin must *NEVER* be withdrawn from a cartridge or insulin pen—this is unsafe and can lead to inaccuracies in insulin dosages.

Table 5.2 Prefilled disposable pen devices

	Prefilled Disposable Pen Devices						**Diabetes Specialist** Nurse Forum UK
Manufacturer	Insulin	Device name	Min-max dose	Dose Increments	Device capacity	Material	Recycle scheme
Novo Nordisk	Fiasp	FlexTouch	1-80 units	1 unit	300 units	Plastic	PenCycle
	Levemir	FlexPen	1-60 units				
	NovoMix 30	FlexPen	1-60 units				
	NovoRapid	FlexPen	1-60 units				
		FlexTouch	1-80 units				
	Tresiba 100 units/ml	FlexTouch	1-80 units				
	Tresiba 200 units/ml	FlexTouch	2-160 units	2 units	600 units		
Sanofi	Admelog**	SoloStar	1-80 units	1 unit	300 units	Plastic	RePen
	Apidra						
	Lantus						
	Trurapi**						
	Toujeo 300 units/ml	SoloStar	1-80 units	1 unit	450 units		
		DoubleStar	2-160 units	2 units	900 units		

(Continued)

Table 5.2 (Contd.)

	Prefilled Disposable Pen Devices						Diabetes Specialist Nurse Forum UK
Eli Lilly	Abasaglar**	KwikPen	1-80 units	1 unit	300 units	Plastic	No
	Humalog 100 units/ml	KwikPen	1-60 units	1 unit	300 units		
		Junior KwikPen	0.5-30 units	0.5 units	300 units		
	Humalog 200 units/ml	KwikPen	1-60 units	1 unit	600 units		
	Humalog Mix25	KwikPen	1-60 units	1 unit	300 units		
	Humalog Mix50						
	Humulin I						
	Humulin M3						
	Lyumjev 100 units/ml	KwikPen	1-60 units	1 unit	300 units		
		Junior KwikPen	0.5-30 units	0.5 units			
	Lyumjev 200 units/ml	KwikPen	1-60 units	1 unit	600 units		
Mylan	Semglee**	Pre-filled pen	1-80 units	1 unit	300 units	Plastic	No

With kind permission from DSN Forum to reproduce – ⏺ https://www.diabetesspecialistnurseforumuk.co.uk/charts

** Biosimilar insulins

Information about the PenCycle scheme can be found at ⏺ https://www.pen-cycle.co.uk

Information about the UK based pilot RePen scheme can be found at ⏺ www.mysanofiinsulin.co.uk/repen

*At the time of publication, insulin levemir (in all device formats) is expected to be discontinued by the end of 2026 and novo-rapid insulin will no longer be available in the flex touch pen device.

Table 5.3 Reusable cartridge pen devices

| Manufacturer | Re-usable Cartridge Pen Devices | | | | | | Diabetes Specialist Nurse Forum UK | |
	Compatible Insulins (3ml cartridges)	Pen device	Min-Max dosage	Dose Increments	Capacity	Colour	Material
Novo Nordisk	Flasp Insulatard Levemir NovoMix 30 NovoRapid Tresiba 100 units/ml	Novopen 6 Smart pen	1-60 units	1 unit	300 units	Blue Silver	Metal & plastic
		Novopen Echo Plus Smart Pen	0.5-30 units	0.5 units	300 units	Teal Red	
Sanofi	Admelog** Apidra Lantus Trurapi**	AllStar PRO	1-80 units	1u nit	300 units	Blue Siver	Plastic
		Junior STAR	0.5-30 units	0.5 units	300 units	Red Blue Silver	

(Continued)

Table 5.3 (Contd.)

	Re-usable Cartridge Pen Devices					Diabetes Specialist Nurse Forum UK	
Eli Lilly	Abasaglar** Humalog 100 units/ml Humalog Mix 25 Humalog Mix 50 Humulin I Humulin M3 Humulin S Lyumjev 100 units/ml	HumaPen Savvio	1-60 units	1 unit	300 units	Blue Graphite Red	Metal
Wockhardt	Porcine Neutral Porcine Isophane Porcine 30/70 Mix	Owen Munford Autopen Classic 1-unit pen	1-21 units	1 unit	300 units	Dark green	Plastic
		Owen Munford Autopen Classic 2-unit pen	2-42 units	2 units	300 units	Dark blue	

With kind permission from DSN Forum to reproduce – ℗ https://www.diabetesspecialistnurseforumuk.co.uk/charts

** Biosimilar insulins

All re-usable cartridge pens can be prescribed via FP10, a spare pen device should always be available in case of loss or breakage.

*At the time of publication, insulin levemir (in all device formats) is expected to be discontinued by the end of 2026

Selecting an insulin regimen

No single regimen is appropriate for all. Important factors to consider that will influence choice include an individual's preference with regard to frequency of injecting, lifestyle factors, including eating habits, physical activity, day-to-day variability, and whether a third party is required to administer the insulin.

Consider the following factors when choosing an insulin regimen:

- Is the person willing and/or able to self-inject (consider cognitive ability, manual dexterity, visual capacity)?
- Does the person eat the same number and type of meals each day?
- Do they have a varied lifestyle involving shift work and erratic mealtimes?
- How often does the person exercise?
- Does the person have a preference for the number of injections per day?
- Would the person require a carer or community nurse to administer the insulin?
- What would be the impact of hypoglycaemia (e.g. do they live alone, are they frail or at risk of falls, are they a frequent or an occupational driver)?
- How motivated is the person to self-monitor blood glucose?
- Is the person able to adjust insulin doses based on self-monitoring of blood glucose?
- Is weight an issue?
- Any other health beliefs/cultural factors to consider?

See also NICE Guidance [NG28].[5]

Reference

1. National Institute for Health and Care Excellence (2015, last updated June 2022). *Type 2 diabetes in adults: management.* NICE guideline [NG28]. Available at: ℜ www.nice.org.uk/guidance/ng28

Practical considerations when starting insulin therapy

Consider the following:
- Factors that influence the choice of insulin regimen, and the benefits and limitations of each regimen
- The delivery device (taking into account manual dexterity/eyesight, etc.)
- Realistic expectations around efficacy (agreeing individual blood glucose targets)
- Explain the action of insulin and timing of injections (especially in relation to meals)
- Concurrent medications (which diabetes-lowering medications need to be stopped)
- Storage of insulin and reconstitution/resuspension
- Safe disposal of sharps
- Injection technique (needle size, changing needles, sharps disposal, site selection, giving an injection, site rotation, identifying and preventing lipohypertrophy)
- Self-monitoring of blood glucose (including interpreting and acting on the results)
- Titrating the insulin dose to achieve agreed blood glucose targets
- Identifying, avoiding, and treating hypoglycaemia (see ➔ Chapter 12)
- Managing insulin and adjusting doses during intercurrent illness ('Sick Day Guidance') (see ➔ Chapter 17)
- Driving, insurance, Driver and Vehicle Licensing Agency (DVLA) guidance, and employment issues (see ➔ Chapter 17 for DVLA advice)
- Impact of physical activity and exercise
- Impact of different foods (especially carbohydrate awareness) and alcohol (see ➔ Chapter 4)
- Issuing insulin passport and insulin safety booklet
- Continuing telephone support and out-of-hours support.

Glycaemic target recommendations
(See ➔ Chapter 7.)

Injection technique

Correct injection technique is crucial to achieve the expected absorption and action of insulin and can affect the safety and efficacy of insulin therapy.

- Insulin storage:
  - Insulin in current use may be stored at room temperature (within expiry date; check the manufacturer's guidance for the length of time the insulin can be stored at room temperature, as this varies across insulins).
  - Avoid direct sunlight and extremes of temperatures, as this can permanently damage the insulin.
  - Unopened insulin should be stored in an area of the refrigerator where freezing is unlikely to occur.
- Resuspension of insulin:
  - Cloudy insulins (e.g. intermediate-acting (NPH) and premixed insulin) must be gently rolled 10 times and inverted 10 times (not shaken) until the crystals go back into suspension and the solution becomes milky white before injecting.
- Needle size, and angle and depth of injection:
  - Insulin is intended to be deposited in the subcutaneous tissue. This is reliably achieved by using a 4 or 5mm needle injected at a 90° angle, with no lifted skinfold.
  - Needles of 4, 5, and 6mm are suitable for all people with diabetes, regardless of age, gender, ethnicity, or body mass index, and there is no clinical reason for recommending needles longer than 6mm.
  - A lifted skinfold should only be considered when using a needle of >6mm or if the person is very slim. The needle should be inserted directly into the skin (not through clothing) at a 90° angle.
- Intramuscular injection of insulin should be avoided, as rapid absorption and serious hypoglycaemia can result.
- Injection sites:
  - The three preferred sites for injection are the abdomen, thighs, and buttocks.
  - If a person chooses to inject into the arm, a 4mm needle is recommended to avoid the risk of intramuscular injection; alternatively, it should be administered by a third party and using a lifted skinfold.
  - Absorption rates differ across these different areas. When using non-analogue insulin, absorption is slowest from the thigh and buttock and fastest from the abdomen.
  - Individuals should be taught an easy-to-follow rotation scheme from the onset of injection therapy.
  - The thigh and buttock are the preferred injection sites when using intermediate-acting (NPH) insulin as the basal insulin, as absorption is slowest from these sites.
  - The abdomen is the preferred site for soluble human insulin, as absorption is fastest there.
  - Premixed insulin (human or analogue) should be given in the abdomen in the morning to increase the speed of absorption of

the rapid- or short-acting insulin to cover post-breakfast glycaemic excursions.
- Premixed insulin should be given in the thigh or buttock before evening meals, as this leads to slower absorption and decreases the risk of nocturnal hypoglycaemia.
- After administering the full dose by fully depressing the plunger, the needle should be left in the skin for at least 10 seconds before withdrawing it to ensure the full dose is given.
- Reusing needles damages the skin tissue and increases the risk of developing lipohypertrophy and should be avoided.
- Massaging the site before or after injection may speed up absorption and is not generally recommended.
- It is important to rotate injection sites to reduce the risk of developing lipohypertrophy—a common problem associated with poor injection technique, affecting as many as 50% of people using insulin in their lifetime.
  - Lipohypertrophy is fatty, rubbery tissue found in the subcutaneous layer that is associated with repeated use of the same injection site and can lead to variable absorption and erratic glycaemic levels. Caution should be exercised when switching injection sites from areas of lipohypertrophy to normal tissue, as this often requires a reduction in the dose of insulin injected.
  - Examination of injection sites should be part of regular review.
- Empty pen devices can be disposed of in the normal household refuse when the needle is removed. Needles and syringes must be disposed of safely in a sharps disposal box—these may be prescribed and collected according to local policy.

Injection technique checklist
- Is a new needle used every time?
- Is the pen device primed to ensure the needle and pen are working correctly with a 2-unit 'air shot'?
- Is the correct-sized needle selected?
- Is insulin stored correctly according to the manufacturer's instructions?
- Is an appropriate area/site on the body being used for injections?
- Before injecting, is the area checked for signs of lumpiness below the skin, so that these areas can be avoided?
- Is a site rotation pattern being followed?
- Are injections being rotated within the chosen site (ensuring each injection is given 1cm away from the last)?
- If the insulin is cloudy, is it being properly resuspended prior to injecting?
- After dialling the required dose, is the needle fully inserted into the skin at an angle of 90°?
- After pressing the dose button, is the needle left *in situ* for a count of 10 to ensure the full dose is delivered?
- Is the needle always safely removed from the pen and disposed of into a sharps bin?

Further information is available from:

- Injection Technique Matters: Best Practice Guideline to Support Correct Injection Technique in Diabetes Care and the Patient Toolkit can be downloaded from: ✍ https://trenddiabetes.online/
- The Forum for Injection Technique (FIT), available at: ✍ https://fit4diabetes.com/

Insulin safety

Given that insulin is such a high-risk medication, it should only be initiated and managed by health care professionals with relevant expertise and training. For an update on insulin safety, access the free e-learning module created by the Primary Care Diabetes Society (available at: ✆ www.diabe tesonthenet.com/cpd-modules/the-six-steps-to-insulin-safety).

Some key safety points to remember

• Insulin doses must be administered by using an insulin syringe or a commercial insulin pen device; intravenous syringes must never be used.
• The term 'units' is used in all contexts; abbreviations such as 'U' or 'IU' must never be used.
• All staff treating people with insulin should always have adequate supplies of insulin syringes and subcutaneous needles.
• An insulin syringe must always be used to measure and prepare insulin for an intravenous infusion.
• A training programme should be in place for all health care staff (including medical staff) expected to prescribe, prepare, and administer insulin.
• Policies and procedures for the preparation and administration of insulin and insulin infusions must be current.

Chapter 6

Continuous subcutaneous insulin infusion

Introduction

Continuous subcutaneous insulin infusion (CSII) is a sophisticated way of delivering insulin, with use of a small, portable pumping device, to which the user is continuously attached. Insulin is delivered via a small, self-inserted subcutaneous cannula.

The insulin pump is programmed by the user, with variable rates of background insulin delivery throughout the day and night (basal rates). It can be altered up to 48 times throughout this period, to match the individual's varying insulin sensitivity as closely as possible.

In addition to basal delivery, the user inputs information into the device's inbuilt bolus calculator, which will then offer advice on how much insulin should be delivered. The bolus dose delivered would accompany carbohydrate intake and/or correct blood glucose levels, to help reach the individual's desired target level of blood glucose.

The first commercially available insulin pump was introduced in the UK in 1976, with advances in the technology escalating rapidly over subsequent decades. Although insulin pump uptake is increasing within the UK, we are behind other European countries in terms of the percentage of those living with type 1 diabetes (T1D) who are on this treatment option. Funding and expertise are limiting factors to uptake. Pump initiation and ongoing support are required by an appropriately trained diabetes specialist team.

Regarding funding, there are two main options, these being self-funding or National Health Service (NHS) funding. The cost of an insulin pump is between £2000 and £3000, with ongoing consumables costing an additional £1500/year. NHS funding became more accessible following issue of the National Institute for Health and Care Excellence (NICE) guidance for T1D in 2004, most recently updated in 2022,[1] and the Technology Appraisal (TA) 151 assessment in 2008.[2] TA assessments are recommendations on the use of new and existing medicines, devices, and treatments within the NHS, but uptake remains unfortunately low. Variability is seen throughout the UK, with some areas being high technology users and other areas being far behind.

More recently, further advances in CSII technology have seen the arrival of hybrid closed-loop systems. These systems allow the pump to use information about the user's blood glucose levels, taken from a real-time continuous glucose monitoring (rT-CGM) sensor, and to self-adjust the basal rates as required.

In December 2023, we saw the release of TA943 guidance[3] supporting the use of closed-loop systems in T1D management with the support of a trained multidisciplinary team experienced in CSII and continuous glucose monitoring in T1D. This advancement and availability of this technology will be life-changing for people with T1D and will be more common practice by the time of publication of this book.

References

1. National Institute for Health and Care Excellence (2015, last updated 2022). *Type 1 diabetes in adults: diagnosis and management.* NICE guideline [NG17]. Available at: ℘ www.nice.org.uk/guidance/ng17

2. National Institute for Health and Care Excellence (2008). *Continuous subcutaneous insulin infusion for the treatment of diabetes mellitus*. Technology appraisal guidance [TA151]. Available at: ⌖ www.nice.org.uk/guidance/ta151

3. National Institute for Health and Care Excellence (2023). *Hybrid closed loop systems for managing blood glucose levels in type 1 diabetes*. Technology appraisal guidance [TA943]. Available at: ⌖ www.nice.org.uk/guidance/ta943

Advantages and disadvantages of continuous subcutaneous insulin infusion

Advantages

- Insulin is absorbed better and delivered more consistently than with a pen.
- Fewer needle injections—especially advantageous for those with needle phobia.
- Flexible insulin delivery (i.e. basal insulin can be ↓ to accommodate unplanned activity and ↑ when unwell with greater ease/immediacy).
- Small incremental insulin changes to delivery can be made—hence more dose precision.
- ↑ patient experience and satisfaction.

Disadvantages

- The user is attached to the device 24/7 and only takes it off for around 1 hour to shower/swim or engage in contact sports.
- Risk of infection if the cannula is not changed with the recommended regularity (every 2–3 days).
- ↑ risk of DKA if pump delivery is interrupted (can occur very quickly in the absence of insulin delivery).
- Practicalities of day-to-day management and use are challenging, particularly when users are new to CSII.
- ↑ cost to the NHS—CSII is a more expensive method of insulin delivery, compared with via pen/injections.

Commencing insulin pump therapy

Things to consider before going ahead:
- NICE guidance should be met with regard to eligible criteria, including the future user undergoing structured education to ensure a solid knowledge base (Dose Adjustment for Normal Eating (DAFNE), a 5-day course covering all aspects of living with T1D).
- Users' expectations should be managed/discussed.
- Care should be taken to discuss the choice of device most appropriate for the individual.

Starting doses

- Basal reduction of 20–25% (e.g. person on 12 units of long-acting insulin/day twice daily; 20% of 24 = 4.8; 24 − 4.8 = 19.2, divided by 24 = 0.8 units/hour). An initial flat basal rate is programmed, adjusting as needed thereafter, depending an individual's requirements.
- Insulin:carbohydrate ratios (e.g. 1 unit of insulin to cover 10g of carbohydrate) and correction bolus (e.g. 1 unit of insulin to lower blood glucose level by 3mmol) as established by the user on their multiple injection regime.

Optimizing control/pump settings

Close follow-up between the specialist health care team and the user is required, with settings being reviewed, alongside pump and blood glucose monitor downloads to guide the necessary changes.

Optimizing settings can be very individual, with some taking much longer to establish their basal settings (along with insulin:carbohydrate ratios and correction factors).

Ongoing, easily accessible support from an experienced team is essential for ongoing success.

Backup plans/troubleshooting

The user always needs access to insulin delivered by a pen device and a clear plan as to the amount to inject in the event of mechanical pump failure. Ensuring that all pump users always have in-date long-acting and rapid-acting insulin available is essential. Users should take plenty of pump supplies, as well as backup pens with them, if travelling/away from home.

All pump companies have 24-hour advice lines for mechanical issues with their devices. The clinical team would be the point of contact if the advice sought is more related to pump settings (i.e. ↑ frequency of hypoglycaemia, heightened blood glucose variability, etc.).

All pump users should be aware of the sick day guidance, and have access to insulin pens, ketone meters, and test strips to minimize the risk of escalation into diabetic ketoacidosis (see ➡ chapter 3, DKA).

Management of CSII when in hospital

Most users are safer remaining on CSII if they remain well enough to self-manage. If, at any point, self-management is not possible, then the pump should be removed, and insulin given by an alternative method (i.e. intravenously) or via a pen device until the person's condition and ability to self-manage return. The pump should be stored in a safe place or sent home with a relative until needed.

For a planned admission/surgical procedure, the user may find it easier to manage the fasting period on CSII, due to the flexibility of insulin delivery.

Suggest CSII discontinuation for major procedures requiring general anaesthesia for >2 hours and use of intravenous insulin instead. When the pump user has recovered and can self-manage, the intravenous insulin should be discontinued 1 hour after the pump has been resited and back in use. This overlapping mitigates hyperglycaemia by ensuring the CSII basal delivery has been established.

In the event of a person needing magnetic resonance imaging or computed tomography scanning (i.e. any radiation exposure), the user should remove their pump. Scans/investigations where the user is disconnected for no longer than 1 hour would not require insulin via an alternative route.

Conclusion

In conclusion, CSII stands as a remarkable milestone in the management of diabetes with the use of sleek, user-friendly devices. CSII empowers individuals to take charge of their diabetes management, refine their blood glucose control, and reduce the risk of complications. Its use and ongoing developments in technology within T1D ensures a brighter future for this community.

Assessment of glycaemia and management of non-urgent hyperglycaemia

Introduction

Studies as far back as the UKPDS[1,2] (type 2 diabetes (T2D)) and DCCT[3] (type 1 diabetes (T1D)) showed a correlation between the development of complications of diabetes and exposure to prolonged raised circulating blood glucose levels.

Indeed, results from the 44-year follow-up of UKPDS[4] showed the important legacy effect of early intensive blood glucose management in the reduction of microvascular complications and improvement in clinical outcomes.

The ACCORD[5] study, however, served to underline that in reducing risk, it is important to balance optimal glycaemic levels with the avoidance of episodes of hypoglycaemia, as both hyper- and hypoglycaemia carry both short- and long-term risk in diabetes (see ➔ Chapter 12).

In the Victorian era, a practice called uroscopy or uronmancy was used, involving the colour, smell, and even taste of urine to make assessments for diabetes. Thankfully there has now been progression from this and the chapter describes how glycaemia can be assessed through capillary blood glucose monitoring (CBGM), HbA1c values, and/or continuous glucose monitoring (CGM).

At all times, it is important to be mindful of ensuring that the person with diabetes and their families and carers have the education and support to enable understanding and self-management. Any desired glycaemic 'targets' need to be individualized, based on a person's life circumstances, including possible multiple long-term conditions, and should be decided only after shared decision-making.

This chapter will also look to discuss the management of non-emergency hyperglycaemia in both T1D and T2D.

For emergency management of hyper- and hypoglycaemia, see ➔ Chapter 12.

References

1. UK Prospective Diabetes Study (UKPDS) Group. Intensive blood-glucose control with sulphonylureas or insulin compared with conventional treatment and risk of complications in patients with type 2 diabetes (UKPDS 33). *The Lancet.* 1998;**352**:837–53.
2. UK Prospective Diabetes Study (UKPDS) Group. Effect of intensive blood-glucose control with metformin on complications in overweight patients with type 2 diabetes (UKPDS 34). *The Lancet.* 1998;**352**:854–65.
3. The Diabetes Control and Complications Trial Research Group. The effect of intensive treatment of diabetes on the development and progression of long-term complications in insulin-dependent diabetes mellitus. *New England Journal of Medicine.* 1993;**329**:977–86.
4. Alder A (2022). *UKPDS perspective, legacy effects and 44-year follow-up data.* Session: S22 UKPDS 44-Year Follow-Up Symposium. Hybrid 58th EASD Annual Meeting. Available at: ✍ www.easd.org/media-centre/#!resources/ukpds-perspective-legacy-effects-and-44-year-follow-up-data
5. Riddle MC. Effects of intensive glucose lowering in the management of patients with type 2 diabetes mellitus in the Action to Control Cardiovascular Risk in Diabetes (ACCORD) trial. *Circulation.* 2010;**122**(8):844–6.

Self-monitoring of capillary blood glucose levels

CBGM allows for assessment of current circulating blood glucose levels.

All people with T1D and certain cohorts of people with T2D should have access to CBGM.[1,2]

Persons with T2D who should be offered CBGM, as suggested by National Institute for Health and Care Excellence (NICE),[2] include the following:

- All individuals treated with insulin
- If there is evidence that a person is experiencing episodes of hypoglycaemia
- If a person is taking oral medication (e.g. a sulfonylurea or postprandial regulator) that may increase their risk of hypoglycaemia
- Where there are Driver and Vehicle Licensing Agency (DVLA) requirements for group 2 drivers (see ➲ Chapter 17)
- If a person is pregnant or planning a pregnancy.

In addition, CBGM may be needed in the shorter term for those:

- Starting treatment with oral or intravenous corticosteroids
- With intercurrent illness causing hyperglycaemia
- With a need to confirm suspected hypoglycaemia.

Most people with type T1D and some with T2D will be using CGM (see ➲ pp. 108–110 in this chapter), but it is vital that these people are still able to check capillary blood glucose levels during times of rapidly changing glucose levels, in case of CGM device failure and as per DVLA regulations for group 2 drivers.

Important considerations

- CBGM should be offered as an integral part of self-management education.
- CBGM skills should be reviewed at least annually, including:
  - How the equipment is maintained/cleaned and correct storage of testing strips (see individual manufacturer's instructions)
  - Ensuring the quality, frequency, and timing of testing are appropriate
  - Provision of support and education to ensure that the person and their family and/or carers can interpret the blood glucose results and know what action to take if they are out with their individualized target levels
  - The impact on the person's quality of life
  - The continued benefit to the person.

Suggested CBGM targets

Capillary blood glucose level targets should always be individualized, based on a person's circumstances and potential coexistence of multiple long-term conditions and/or frailty.

- The general target range is 4–9mmol/L, with pre-meal targets of 4–7mmol/L and post-meal targets of <9mmol/L.
- In pregnancy, NICE glucose targets are lower,[3] with a desired fasting glucose level of <5.7mmol/L, 1-hour postprandial glucose level of

<7.8mmol/L, and 2-hour postprandial level of <6.4mmol/L (see Chapter 15).

- For those with moderate or severe frailty, suggested targets are 6.7–11.1mmol/L.[4]

References

1. National Institute for Health and Care Excellence (2015, last updated 2022). *Type 1 diabetes in adults: diagnosis and management*. NICE guideline [NG17]. Available at: www.nice.org.uk/guidance/ng17
2. National Institute for Health and Care Excellence (2015, last updated 2022). *Type 2 diabetes in adults: management*. NICE guideline [NG28]. Available at: www.nice.org.uk/guidance/ng28
3. National Institute for Health and Care Excellence (2015, last updated 2020). *Diabetes in pregnancy: management from preconception to the postnatal period*. NICE guideline [NG3]. Available at: www.nice.org.uk/guidance/ng3
4. Sinclair A, Gallagher A (2019). *Managing frailty and associated comorbidities in older adults with diabetes: Position Statement on behalf of the Association of British Clinical Diabetologists (ABCD)*. Available at: https://abcd.care/sites/default/files/site_uploads/Resources/Position-Papers/ABCD-Position-Paper-Frailty.pdf

HbA1c

Haemoglobin A1c (HbA1c), or glycosylated HbA1c, is a blood test to determine the amount of glucose in the circulating blood over time (the preceding 3 months). The laboratory test is performed on a venous sample of blood and estimates the amount of glucose that has adhered to haemoglobin in a red blood cell (erythrocyte). The higher the level of glucose in the circulating blood, the more it will 'stick' to the haemoglobin and the higher the number in the HbA1c value.

Measurement is calculated by using methods calibrated according to International Federation of Clinical Chemistry (IFCC) standardization.

HbA1c is used in the diagnosis of T2D where onset is often insidious, and in assessing for glycaemia to support shared decision-making in optimal management.

Circumstances when HbA1c is not suitable for the diagnosis of diabetes include:
- All children and young people
- Suspected T1D (see ➔ Chapter 3)
- High risk and acutely ill (e.g. requiring hospital admission)
- When taking medication that may cause glucose levels to rise rapidly (e.g. steroids, immune checkpoint inhibitors)
- Acute pancreatic damage, including pancreatic surgery
- Pregnancy.

Circumstances when HbA1c is not suitable for the diagnosis or monitoring of diabetes include:
- Presence of genetic, haematological, and illness-related factors that influence HbA1c and its measurement
- In conditions associated with ↑ red blood cell turnover such as:
  - Sickle cell disease
  - Glucose-6-phosphate dehydrogenase deficiency
  - Haemodialysis
  - Recent blood loss or transfusion
  - Erythropoietin therapy.
- HbA1c is also less reliable than blood glucose measurement in other conditions such as:
  - Post-partum
  - HIV treated with certain medications
  - Iron deficiency anaemia
  - Persons on dialysis.

If HbA1c monitoring is invalid because of disturbed erythrocyte turnover or abnormal haemoglobin type, assessment of glycaemia can be performed via one of the following:
- Quality-controlled plasma glucose profiles
- Total glycated haemoglobin estimation (if abnormal haemoglobin)
- Fructosamine estimation.

Measurement interval of HbA1c, as suggested by NICE

Type 1 diabetes
- Every 3–6 months.[1]

Type 2 diabetes
- Every 3–6 months (tailored to individual needs) until HbA1c is stable on unchanging therapy when it may then be measured every 6 months.[2]

Targets

As for CBGM and CGM, targets for HbA1c attainment must always be individualized (see Fig. 7.1) and agreed with the person with diabetes and, where appropriate, with family and carers.[3]

Type 1 diabetes
NICE advocates for a target HbA1c level of 48mmol/mol but advises that this should be in the absence of problematic hypoglycaemia. If hypoglycaemia is frequent, then the HbA1c target needs to be relaxed, with consideration of a person's daily activities, aspirations, and likelihood of complications.[1]

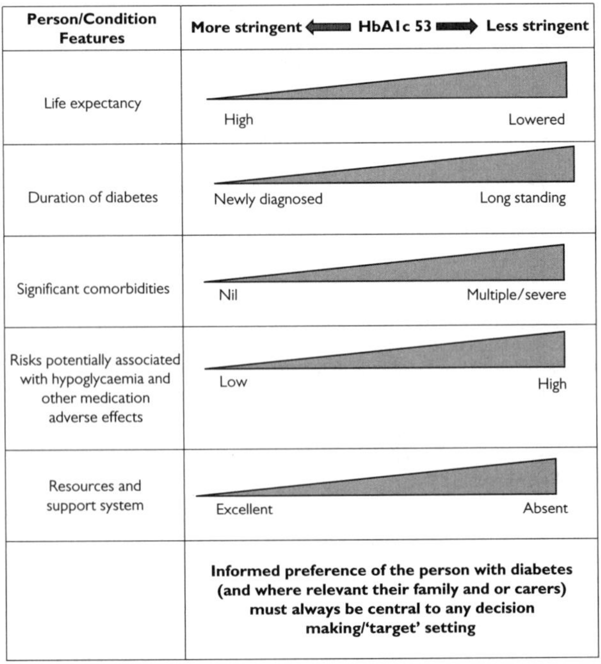

Person/Condition Features	More stringent ◄■■■ HbA1c 53 ■■■► Less stringent	
Life expectancy	High	Lowered
Duration of diabetes	Newly diagnosed	Long standing
Significant comorbidities	Nil	Multiple/severe
Risks potentially associated with hypoglycaemia and other medication adverse effects	Low	High
Resources and support system	Excellent	Absent
	Informed preference of the person with diabetes (and where relevant their family and or carers) must always be central to any decision making/'target' setting	

Fig. 7.1 Individualising glycaemic targets for people living with diabetes.

Type 2 diabetes
- If managed either by lifestyle and diet or by lifestyle and diet combined with a single medication not associated with hypoglycaemia, aim for an HbA1c level of 48mmol/mol or less.
- For adults with T2D on a medication associated with hypoglycaemia, the target HbA1c is <53mmol/mol.[2]

Consideration of relaxation of the target HbA1c level is required for people who are older or more frail if (see Table 7.1):
- They are unlikely to achieve longer-term risk reduction benefits (e.g. people with reduced life expectancy)
- Tight blood glucose control would put the person at high risk if they develop hypoglycaemia (e.g. if they are at risk of falling, they have impaired awareness of hypoglycaemia, or they drive or operate machinery as part of their job)
- Intensive management would not be appropriate (e.g. if they have significant comorbidities or are on an end-of-life pathway).

Table 7.1 Suggested individualized glucose targets in persons living with frailty

Moderate frailty	• >2 comorbidities	• HbA1c <64mmol/mol
	• Reduced life expectancy	• FPG 6.0–8.3mmol/L
Severe frailty	• Significant comorbidity, functional deficits, and limited independence	• HbA1c <69mmol/mol
	• Markedly reduced life expectancy	• FPG 7.0–10.0mmol/L

℘ https://link.springer.com/article/10.1007/s13300-021-01035-9/tables/3

For women who are trying to conceive, NICE suggests a target HbA1c value of <48mmol/mol[4] (see ➲ Chapter 14).

References

1. National Institute for Health and Care Excellence (2015, last updated 2022). *Type 1 diabetes in adults: diagnosis and management.* NICE guideline [NG17]. Available at: ℘ www.nice.org.uk/guidance/ng17
2. National Institute for Health and Care Excellence (2015, last updated 2022). *Type 2 diabetes in adults: management.* NICE guideline [NG28]. Available at: ℘ www.nice.org.uk/guidance/ng28
3. Davies MJ, Aroda VR, Collins BS, *et al.* Management of hyperglycaemia in type 2 diabetes, 2022. A consensus report by the American Diabetes Association (ADA) and the European Association for the Study of Diabetes (EASD). *Diabetologia.* 2022;**65**:1925–66. Available at: ℘ https://diabetesjournals.org/care/issue/46/Supplement_1
4. National Institute for Health and Care Excellence (2015, last updated 2020). *Diabetes in pregnancy: management from preconception to the postnatal period.* NICE guideline [NG3]. Available at: ℘ www.nice.org.uk/guidance/ng3

Continuous glucose monitoring

Both real-time CGM (rtCGM) and intermittently scanned CGM (isCGM) are methods of measuring glucose levels from interstitial fluid (fluid between cells), without the need for routine capillary blood glucose testing.

rtCGM records glucose levels continuously throughout the day and night, providing both real-time and predictive glucose data.

A small sensor is worn, usually on the arm or abdomen, which inputs interstitial glucose data continually via Bluetooth to the wearer's smart device.

People using a reader not linked to a smart device may need to intermittently scan their sensor. To obtain sufficient data for a complete glucose profile, the sensor must be scanned at least every 8 hours, although optimally >6 times a day.

There are various CGM systems available—some are available in primary care, but some, particularly those that work with insulin pumps or enable closed-loop systems, may only be available via the NHS supply chain through specialist secondary care services.

Potential benefits

- Reduction in finger prick testing.
- Trend arrows can aid in safe and effective adjustments of treatment to avoid hypo- and hyperglycaemia.
- Alarms can be set to alert the user to potential hypo- and hyperglycaemic events.
- Patterns in glucose variation can be identified.
- Easier and less invasive identification of night-time hypoglycaemia.
- Can enhance self-management and user engagement.
- Carers and parents can access readings and data.
- Generates a full 24-hour glycaemic picture.
- Studies show ↑ time in glucose target range and a potentially improved HbA1c, thus reducing the risk of long-term diabetes complications.
- Positive impact on quality of life.
- Data can be uploaded to share online with health care professionals (HCPs) via compatible systems (subject to local data-sharing agreements), enabling more effective consultations and remote reviews.
- Studies in people with T1D show cost-effectiveness, compared with finger prick testing.
- Larger text displays and spoken glucose readings are possible for those with visual impairment.

Possible disadvantages

- Data overload can confuse or worry some users.
- Interstitial fluid glucose time lag—thus, a fingerpick test is still required in periods of rapidly changing glucose levels.
- Possible sensor problems relating to skin irritation or adhesive failure.
- Group 2 drivers currently still need to check capillary blood glucose levels for driving.[1]

Who is eligible?

It is important that all HCPs are aware of their contemporaneous local and national guidance on eligibility criteria.

Current guidance supports eligibility to all persons with T1D.[2]

In T2D NICE advise that people that be considered are those on multiple daily doses of insulin if any of the following apply:[3]

- Recurrent hypoglycaemia or severe hypoglycaemia
- Impaired hypoglycaemia awareness
- A condition or disability (including a learning disability or cognitive impairment) that means the user cannot self-monitor capillary blood glucose levels but can use a CGM device.
- The person would otherwise be advised to self-monitor capillary glucose at least eight times a day.
- The person is insulin-treated and would otherwise need help from a care worker or healthcare professional to monitor their blood glucose levels
- Pregnant women who are on insulin therapy but who do not have T1D if they have:
  - Problematic severe hypoglycaemia (with or without impaired awareness of hypoglycaemia)
  - Unstable blood glucose levels that are causing concern despite efforts to optimize glycaemic control.

Important considerations

Blood glucose vs interstitial fluid

- Blood glucose and interstitial glucose levels are closely related, but not identical.
- There is a time lag of ~2–4 minutes (depending on which device is used) for glucose levels measured from the interstitial fluid.
- Therefore, in times of rapidly changing blood glucose levels (e.g. after eating or exercise), or when there are symptoms of hypoglycaemia, a finger prick blood glucose measurement is indicated.

NB people with T1D will also still need access to a means of testing for ketones.

Initiation: top tips

- Ensure shared decision-making to identify the most appropriate device.
- Download the device's compatible mobile app.
- If a smart device is not available, arrange for a compatible reader before fitting.
- See manufacturers' specific guidance on how to apply the sensor.
- Set low and high alarms based on individualized target glycaemic range.
- Signpost the user and/or their family and carers to appropriate education to enable self-management.
- Provide information on future need for capillary glucose testing, driving, etc.
- Consider linking to the device's cloud-based system (depending on local data-sharing guidelines), so that data can be shared from the person's own account to the HCPs clinic account.
- Ensure the person understands when their data will be reviewed.
- Arrange for timely review/follow-up.

Time in range

With the advent of CGM, there is now the ability to review glucose variability across time spans. Time in range (TIR) is the term given to the portion of time as a percentage that a person with diabetes spends with glucose readings in each of the three defined glucose ranges:

- Desired TIR 3.9–10mmol/L
- Time below range <3.8mmol/L
- Time above range >10.0mmol/L.

The consensus is for 70% TIR,[4] but as with all other glycaemic targets in diabetes, there are different targets for women in pregnancy and people living with moderate or severe frailty (see ➲ pp. 111–113).

For every 10% increase in TIR, there is 40% risk reduction in microalbuminuria and 64% reduction in retinopathy.[4]

Reviewing the data: top tips

- Respect the person's data and avoid negative language.
- Work in collaboration.
- Look to reduce time below range (see ➲ Chapter 12 on hypoglycaemia).
- Look to minimize time above range (see ➲ pp. 115–116 in this chapter).

Common areas causing variability and/or reduced TIR

- Limited sensor glucose data.
- Unsuitable TIR targets.
- Incorrect timing of insulin.
- Incorrect dose of insulin.
- Under-reacting to glucose levels.
- Overreacting to glucose levels.
- Overtreating hypoglycaemia.
- Poor injection technique, including injecting into areas of lipohypertrophy (see ➲ Chapter 5).

Resources

- The ABCD Diabetes Technology Network: resources and education, including videos and modules for HCPs and people with diabetes. Available at: ✍ https://abcd.care/abcd-diabetes-technology-network
- See also manufacturers' websites for advice on device use. (These websites include both HCP and user educational resources and academies to boost knowledge and understanding around data interpretation.)
- Primary Care Diabetes Society CGM Modules available at ✍ https://diabetesonthenet.com/cpd-modules/

Time in ranges:
targets for people with type 1 or type 2 diabetes

Thinking about individualised targets

A person with **HbA1c of 53–63 mmol/mol (7.0–7.9%)** will see on average a **4 mmol/mol (0.4%) reduction** with each **10% (2 h 24 min) increase in TIR**

A person with **HbA1c of ≥64 mmol/mol (≥8.0%)** can see on average a 11 mmol/mol (1.0%) reduction in HbA1c with each **10% (2 h 24 min) increase in TIR**

A **10% (2 h 24 min) decrease in TAR** can be associated on average with a **reduction in HbA1c of approx 7 mmol/mol (0.6%)**

For **age <25 years with type 1 diabetes, if the HbA1c goal is 58 mmol/mol (7.5%), set TIR target to approx 60%**

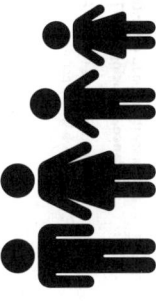

Very high (>13.9 mmol/l)	Level 2 hyperglycaemia	<5% <1 h 12 min
High (10.0–13.9 mmol/l)	Level 1 hyperglycaemia	<25%* <6 h
Target range (3.9–10.0 mmol/l)		>70% >16 h 48 min
Low (<3.9 mmol/l)	Level 1 hyperglycaemia	<4% <1 h*
Very low (<3.0 mmol/l)	Level 2 hyperglycaemia	<1% <15 min

Glucose level (mmol/L)

* Readings >13.9 mmol/l are also included in the <25% target
Readings <3.0 mmol/l are also included in the <4% target

Time in Range:
targets for older people and those at high-risk of hypoglycaemia

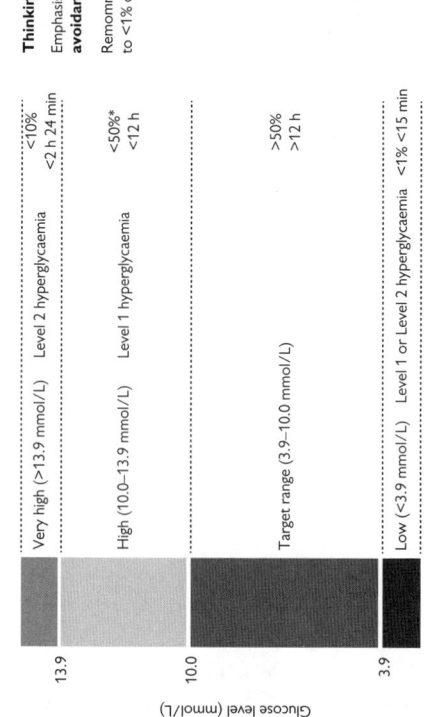

Thinking about individualised targets

Emphasise the need to **prioritise hypoglycaemia avoidance, reducing the %TBR <3.9 mmol/L**

Recommendation is to keep %TBR <3.9 mmol/L to <1% or 15 min per day

HIGH RISK

Very high (>13.9 mmol/L)   Level 2 hyperglycaemia   <10%
<2 h 24 min

High (10.0–13.9 mmol/L)   Level 1 hyperglycaemia   <50%*
<12 h

Target range (3.9–10.0 mmol/L)   >50%
>12 h

Low (<3.9 mmol/L)   Level 1 or Level 2 hyperglycaemia   <1% <15 min

Glucose level (mmol/L)

13.9

10.0

3.9

* Readings >13.9 mmol/L are also included in the <50% target

Time in Range:
targets for women with type 1 diabetes who are pregnant*

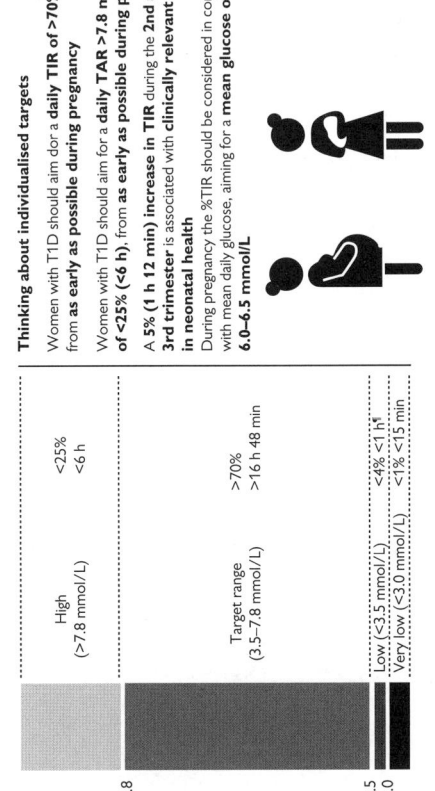

Thinking about individualised targets

Women with T1D should aim dor a **daily TIR of >70% (16 h 48 min)** from **as early as possible during pregnancy**

Women with T1D should aim for a **daily TAR >7.8 mmol/L of <25% (<6 h)**, from **as early as possible during pregnancy**

A **5% (1 h 12 min) increase in TIR** during the **2nd and early 3rd trimester** is associated with **clinically relevant improvements in neonatal health**

During pregnancy the %TIR should be considered in conjunction with mean daily glucose, aiming for a **mean glucose of 6.0–6.5 mmol/L**

High
(>7.8 mmol/L)   <25%
                       <6 h

Target range
(3.5–7.8 mmol/L)   >70%
                       >16 h 48 min

7.8

Low (<3.5 mmol/L)   <4% <1 h¶
Very low (<3.0 mmol/L) <1% <15 min

3.5
3.0

Glucose level (mmol/L)

* %TIR, %TBR and %TAR are based on limited evidence. More research is needed.
¶ Readings <3.0 mmol/L are also included in the <4% target

References

1. Driver and Vehicle Licensing Agency (2022). *Assessing fitness to drive: a guide for medical professionals*. Available at: ⅍ https://assets.publishing.service.gov.uk/government/uploads/system/uploads/attachment_data/file/1084397/assessing-fitness-to-drive-may-2022.pdf
2. National Institute for Health and Care Excellence (2015, last updated 2022). *Type 1 diabetes in adults: diagnosis and management*. NICE guideline [NG17]. Available at: ⅍ www.nice.org.uk/guidance/ng17
3. National Institute for Health and Care Excellence (2015, last updated 2022). *Type 2 diabetes in adults: management*. NICE guideline [NG28]. Available at: ⅍ www.nice.org.uk/guidance/ng28
4. Wilmott EG, Lumb A, Hammond P, *et al.* (2020). *Time in range: a best practice guide for UK diabetes healthcare professionals in the context of the COVID-19 global pandemic*. Available at: ⅍ https://onlinelibrary.wiley.com/doi/full/10.1111/dme.14433

How to manage non-emergency hyperglycaemia

For persons failing to reach their individualized glucose targets, then a full holistic review is indicated.

It is imperative that the HCP understands the challenges faced by people living with diabetes and the burden this can add to daily life (see ➲ Chapter 8).

Education for diabetes self-management should be offered at diagnosis and should be fundamental to all consultations throughout the diabetes journey of person, so to empower confident self-care in diabetes. This includes signposting to resources and possible peer support.

It is important to avoid being judgemental and affording blame. The principles outlined in The Language Matters Diabetes[1] need to be pivotal to the interactions between the HCP and the person with diabetes and/or their families and carers.

This section of the book will discuss medication approaches to achieving desired glucose levels, but this absolutely needs to be done hand in hand with education, review of emotional and mental well-being, and consideration of a person's life circumstances, health beliefs, and informed choices.

Type 1 diabetes

Possible causes of hyperglycaemia include:
- Insufficient/missed insulin
- Overtreatment of any episodes of hypoglycaemia
- Incorrect injection technique, including injecting into areas of lipohypertrophy
- Dietary factors
- Less activity/exercise than normal
- Underlying illness/infection
- Change in activities of daily living
- Sleep disturbance
- Stress
- Hormonal changes
- New medications (e.g. steroids).

Management may include:
- Titration of insulin doses
- Strategies to ensure no missed insulin/use of smart insulin pens
- Avoidance and correct management of hypoglycaemia
- Where appropriate, correct injection technique or use of insulin pump therapy (see ➲ Chapter 5)
- Review of diet/carbohydrate counting (see ➲ Chapter 4)
- Treatment of any underlying illness/infection as appropriate
- Support with mental and emotional well-being (see ➲ Chapter 8)
- Promotion of optimal sleeping patterns
- Checking for ketones (see ➲ Chapter 3).

Type 2 diabetes

Possible causes of hyperglycaemia include:
- Dietary factors
- Less activity/exercise than normal
- Weight gain—increasing insulin resistance
- Change in activities of daily living
- Natural progression of diabetes/deterioration in β-cell function
- Anti-hyperglycaemic medication not taken as prescribed/missed medication
- New medications (e.g. steroids, antipsychotics)
- Underlying illness/infection
- Disturbance in sleep
- Stress
- Hormonal changes
- Pancreatic cancer (see ➲ Chapter 1)
- For persons using insulin:
  - Insufficient/missed insulin
  - Overtreatment of hypoglycaemia (this would also be for persons taking a sulfonylurea or postprandial regulator)
  - Incorrect injection technique, including injecting into areas of lipohypertrophy.

Management may include:
- Weight optimisation strategies
- Dietary review
- Increase in activity/exercise levels
- Promotion of optimal sleeping patterns
- Support with emotional and mental well-being
- Treatment of any underlying illness/infection
- If feasible, avoidance of medication that may induce hyperglycaemia
- Review of medication regime, including advice on how medications should be taken
- Excluding any possible pancreatic pathology as per local guidance
- Escalating oral/injectable therapies as per local, national, and international guidance[2,3]
- Promoting avoidance of, and correct management for, any episodes of hypoglycaemia
- For persons taking insulin, titrating doses depending on glucose levels, and promoting good injection technique and strategies to avoid missed doses/inappropriate timing of injections.

References

1. NHS England (2023). *Language matters: language and diabetes.* Available at: ℘ www.england.nhs.uk/long-read/language-matters-language-and-diabetes
2. National Institute for Health and Care Excellence (2015, last updated 2022). *Type 1 diabetes in adults: diagnosis and management.* NICE guideline [NG17]. Available at: ℘ www.nice.org.uk/guidance/ng17
3. National Institute for Health and Care Excellence (2015, last updated 2022). *Type 2 diabetes in adults: management.* NICE guideline [NG28]. Available at: ℘ www.nice.org.uk/guidance/ng28

Psychological issues in people living with diabetes

Introduction

Managing a long-term condition is demanding, as diabetes is often likened to a person needing to beat their own heart. It is a condition that requires constant attention and care, and it can be overwhelming. The long-term nature of diabetes also means that the relationship between health care professionals (HCPs) working in this field and the people they support can feel more involved than in other conditions. This chapter will explore the psychological aspects of managing diabetes, the prevalence of psychological distress among people living with diabetes, and how HCPs can better support those living with this condition.

Prevalence and causes of common psychological issues in people living with diabetes

- Depression and anxiety are 50% more prevalent in people living with diabetes.[1]
- Suicidal intent is higher in people living with diabetes.[2]
- Eating disorders are three times more likely in young people living with T1D.[3]

In almost every measurable metric of mental health, it is reliably observed that people living with diabetes experience worse psychological health than people who do not live with chronic conditions. There are many reasons for this.

Firstly, diabetes management introduces a host of burdens that add to existing stress levels. These include general long-term condition burdens, such as organizing medications, adaptations to lifestyle, and frequent interactions with a health system that may not always feel helpful, and diabetes-specific burdens in the form of blood glucose monitoring, carbohydrate counting, dealing with hypoglycaemic episodes, and managing an inherently unstable condition. As well as these practical burdens, people with diabetes may worry more about their long-term health and mortality and will frequently encounter stigma.[4]

These management burdens alone may be enough to push a person past the point of routine stress and into longer-standing psychological distress issues. However, many people with diabetes will also possess personal vulnerabilities that also ↑ their likelihood of developing significant psychological distress. These vulnerabilities may include having experienced adverse childhood events (e.g. abuse, neglect), insecure attachment to parents and/or caregivers, neurodevelopmental issues such as autism or attention-deficit/hyperactivity disorder (ADHD), experiences of deprivation and discrimination, and having psychological issues that predate the diagnosis of diabetes.

Once psychological distress is established, it negatively impacts diabetes management through ↓ motivation, ↑ stress hormones, and changes in behaviour around diabetes self-management (e.g. ignoring high levels or impulsive 'rage' bolusing). This results in erratic blood glucose levels, which can further ↑ psychological distress through direct effects of glycaemia on mood, ↑ incidence of self-criticism and anxiety about the future, and ↑ incidence of diabetes complications that cause further decline in mood (depicted in Fig. 8.1).[5,6]

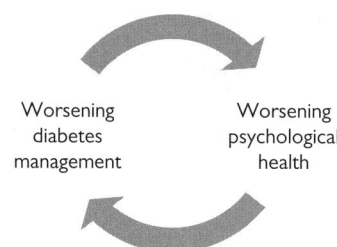

Fig. 8.1 Continuous cycle of increasing psychological distress.

Sadly, the majority of people struggle to access psychological support. This is partly due to diagnostic overshadowing where issues such as depression may be misinterpreted as being part of the normal experience of living with diabetes. It may also be the case that some people with diabetes already feel distressed by the demands of living with a chronic condition and are reluctant to recognize that their mental health may also need attention and support. Furthermore, many people with diabetes who have sought mental health support from generic mental health services may have had the experience of working with a practitioner who does not understand the demands and stresses of living with diabetes, thereby causing the person to feel unheard and potentially rejected. In any case, studies consistently demonstrate that a large proportion of people living with diabetes also live with unmet psychological needs, which have profound negative effects on their quality of life and future health outcomes. Unmet psychological needs will also negatively impact family support systems through ↑ conflict and ↑ carer burden, and they have a profoundly negative effect across the entire health system.

Health economic analysis[7] demonstrated that people living with type 2 diabetes (T2D) and mental health issues have, on average, 50% higher cost of care than those people without mental health issues. ↑ costs come in the form of higher rates of comorbidities (e.g. long-term complications) but are also felt immediately in the form of need for more frequent contact, missed appointments, and ↑ emergency care usage. Mental health issues are also a key predictor of repeat diabetic ketoacidosis (DKA) admissions in people living with type 1 diabetes (T1D).[8]

References

1. Rotella F, Mannucci E. Diabetes mellitus as a risk factor for depression. A meta-analysis of longitudinal studies. *Diabetes Research and Clinical Practice*. 2013;**99**:98–104.
2. Elamoshy RB. Risk of depression and suicidality among diabetic patients: a systematic review and meta-analysis. *Journal of Clinical Medicine*. 2018;**7**(11):445.
3. Hanlan ME, Griffith J, Patel N, Jaser SS. Eating disorders and disordered eating in type 1 diabetes: prevalence, screening, and treatment options. *Current Diabetes Reports*. 2013;**13**:909–16.
4. Embick R, Jackson M, Stewart R. The impact of stigma on the management of type 1 diabetes: a systematic review. *Diabetic Medicine*. 2024;**41**(4):e15299.
5. Hessler DM, Fisher L, Polonsky WH, *et al*. Diabetes distress is linked with worsening diabetes management over time in adults with type 1 diabetes. *Diabetic Medicine*. 2017;**34**(9):1228–34.

6. Fisher L, Glasgow RE, Strycker LA. The relationship between diabetes distress and clinical depression with glycemic control among patients with type 2 diabetes. *Diabetes Care*. 2010;**33**(5):1034–6.
7. Hex N, Bartlett C, Wright D, Taylor M, Varley DJ. Estimating the current and future costs of type 1 and type 2 diabetes in the UK, including direct health costs and indirect societal and productivity costs. *Diabetic Medicine*. 2012;**29**(7):855–62.
8. Allcock B, Stewart R, Jackson M. Psychosocial factors associated with repeat diabetic ketoacidosis in people living with type 1 diabetes: a systematic review. *Diabetic Medicine*. 2022;**39**(1):e14663.

Diabetes-specific psychological issues

Because of the unique interaction between psychological well-being and self-management, people with diabetes are also at risk of developing specific psychological issues that are only related to living with diabetes. While many of these issues cannot be found in diagnostic manuals of psychological distress, the impact that they have on the person who experiences them is certainly detrimental and, at times, profoundly damaging. Common diabetes-specific issues are listed below in Table 8.1. All these issues can be experienced individually or in conjunction with other psychological issues, with severity ranging from slightly concerning to life-threatening.

Table 8.1 Common diabetes-specific psychological issues

Issue	Definition	Common symptoms
Diabetes distress	Negative relationship with diabetes experienced in multiple areas of life (e.g. powerlessness, management distress, stigma) *Can be assessed by using measures such as PAID or DDS (see ◗ Further reading, p. 124)*	• Feelings of failure about diabetes management • Self-blame and judgement • Feeling controlled by diabetes • Resenting diabetes care tasks
Diabetes burnout	Reaching a point of emotional exhaustion with diabetes where self-management tasks feel overwhelming and, as a result, are reduced or ceased	• High diabetes distress • Reduced diabetes self-care behaviours • Feeling numb or uncaring towards diabetes
Fear of hypoglycaemia	An intense fear of hypoglycaemia accompanied by a range of avoidance behaviours	• Deliberately running blood glucose levels higher than recommended • Obsessively checking blood glucose levels • Avoidance of glucose-lowering activities (e.g. exercise)
Hyperglycaemia aversion	An obsessive need to keep blood glucose at the lowest possible level, to the detriment of quality of life	• Obsessively checking blood glucose levels • Frequently taking small bolus doses • Excessive exercise • Dietary restriction

(Continued)

Table 8.1 (Contd.)

Issue	Definition	Common symptoms
Needle phobia	An intense fear of needles accompanied by a range of avoidance behaviours	• Inability to self-inject insulin • Taking an extremely long time to self-inject insulin • Avoidance of blood tests/ vaccinations
Type 1 disordered eating (T1DE—previously referred to as 'diabulimia')	Disturbance in perception of weight/ shape and fear of weight gain, AND deliberate omission or manipulation of insulin for the purposes of weight loss or control *Can be assessed using measures such as DEPS-R (see ➲ Further reading, p. 124)*	• High HbA1c • Repeated DKA admissions • Concealment behaviours (e.g. switching off CGM, pretending to inject, avoiding diabetes care appointments)

PAID, Problem Areas In Diabetes Questionnaire; DDS, Diabetes Distress Scale; DEPS-R, Disordered Eating Problem Survey—revised; DKA, diabetic ketoacidosis; CGM, continuous glucose monitoring.

Instant psychological skills for diabetes nurses

Some people living with diabetes may exhibit very clear psychological issues or will willingly disclose them, whereas others may be unaware of, or unable to communicate about, the issues they experience. It is imperative that the diabetes nurse is familiar with these issues and the signs with which a person may be struggling. Discussing psychological issues may feel challenging at first, but there are many ways in which this part of practice can be developed without significant amounts of additional work or training.

Some simple strategies to help develop skills in this area are listed in Box 8.1.

Box 8.1 Instant psychological skills for diabetes nurses

• Build a relationship—taking the time to find out a little about the person's life, goals, and values will have an enormous impact on your ability to build a therapeutic relationship with them.
• Psychological care needs to be embedded into team routines—regularly consider psychological aspects of care in discussions and include them in your paperwork.
• Think about your own well-being—if you are experiencing high stress, compassion fatigue, or burnout, you will be less attuned to the needs of the people around you.

Box 8.1 (*Contd.*)

- Ask the magic question—'what's one thing about your diabetes that's really getting to you at the moment?' This will communicate that you're open to hearing about a person's stresses and worries without inviting them to offload everything on to you.
- Active listening—remember to use open questions and use your body language to convey listening and connection.
- Normalize, but don't minimize—managing diabetes is hard. Even people who have been living with it for the longest time need to vent about it sometimes.
- Investigate your supports—find out what supports you may be able to signpost to or use. These could include local health psychology teams, community programmes, or third-sector supports. If your team has access to a diabetes psychologist, it is likely that they will be able to provide you with psychological skills training and ongoing supervision to enhance your practice.
- Avoid fear-based approaches—giving lectures on risks of complications is rarely effective and risks breaking down relationships between you and the person with diabetes. Similarly, the language used in consultations can be profoundly impactful—see the Language Matters[1] document for further guidance on this.
- Seek feedback—regularly check in with the people who use your service to find out what is going well and what could be improved. You could also ask a colleague to observe your practice and provide feedback.

Reference

1. NHS England (2023). *Language matters: language and diabetes*. Available at: ℅ www.england.nhs. uk/long-read/language-matters-language-and-diabetes

Conclusion

Psychological distress is the most common complication of living with diabetes that there is. However, despite there being consistently high levels of psychological distress recorded in populations of people living with diabetes, it remains overwhelmingly the case that support is difficult to access, particularly when the person is experiencing issues that are specific to living with diabetes. Psychological well-being needs to be the business of the whole diabetes team, and diabetes nurses are uniquely placed to be able to identify needs and to support people because of their long-term relationships with people living with diabetes. Developing skills and knowledge in this area can help to provide better support and achieve better outcomes.

Further reading

Diabetes Distress Scale (DDS-17). Available at: ℜ https://professional.diabetes.org/sites/default/files/media/ada_mental_health_toolkit_questionnaires.pdf

Eating Disorder Screening (DEPS-R Scale). Available at: ℜ https://clinicalexcellence.qld.gov.au/sites/default/files/docs/priority-area/clinical-engagement/networks/diab/diabetes-deps-r-scale.pdf

Problem Areas In Diabetes (PAID) Scale. Available at: ℜ https://professional.diabetes.org/sites/default/files/media/ada_mental_health_toolkit_questionnaires.pdf

Ongoing care for people with diabetes

Introduction

This brief chapter outlines the gold standards of care that a person living with diabetes should expect from their health care team each year.

This leads into Chapters 10 and 11, which will dive deeper into the bespoke prevention and management of both macro- and microvascular complications of diabetes.

Through regular education, monitoring, and review, it is important to deliver holistic care, which aims to ensure optimal emotional and physical well-being/outcomes for the person with diabetes.

It is also important to consider, where appropriate, the care of family members and/or carers supporting the person with diabetes.

Overwhelming research and real-world evidence underline the need for regular review and individualized target attainment in looking to prevent, and/or delay, any progression of possible long-term complications of diabetes, which include:

- Cardiovascular disease
- Heart failure
- Neuropathy
- Retinopathy
- Nephropathy
- Sexual health dysfunction
- Autonomic neuropathy
- Emotional distress.

Regular review and contemporaneous education also support for a reduction in short-term complications of diabetes, which include the risks from significant hyperglycaemia such as diabetic ketoacidosis and hyperosmolar hyperglycaemic state and from hypoglycaemia (see ➜ Chapter 12).

Diabetes UK promotes the importance of access to the following 'Health Care Essentials' for everyone living with diabetes, on at least an annual basis or more frequently as required/indicated:

- Ensuring the diagnosis is correct (see ➜ Chapter 1)
- Offer of diabetes education, including options for face-to-face, digital, and peer support (see ➜ Chapters 2 and 3)
- Appropriate lifestyle advice, including diet, activity, sleep, and smoking cessation as indicated
- For people with type 2 diabetes, look to the feasibility of a remission pathway (see ➜ Chapter 2)
- Blood pressure measurement and target attainment (see ➜ Chapter 10)
- Lipids measurement and target attainment (see ➜ Chapter 10)
- Measurement and target attainment for glycaemic levels. This is normally by using a HbA1c value, but for some people, this may also include review of capillary blood glucose monitoring values or review of continuous glucose monitoring data, including time in range (see ➜ Chapter 7)
- Blood tests (estimated glomerular filtration rate and urea and electrolytes) and measurement of urine albumin-to-creatinine ratio as part of assessment for, and management of, any nephropathy (see ➜ Chapter 11)

- A review of weight and body mass index. People who are overweight should be supported to lose weight through lifestyle advice and signposting to local weight management services, which would ideally include review by a dietitian (see ➲ Chapter 4)
- Retinal screening—carried out by an optometrist, as per the national screening protocol (see ➲ Chapter 11)
- Foot examination and appropriate footcare advice (see ➲ Chapter 11)
- Support with any sexual health concerns/dysfunction (see ➲ Chapters 11 and 14)
- Screening for, and/or review of, any potential emotional well-being and mental health needs (see ➲ Chapter 8)
- For people with type 1 diabetes, measurement of thyroid levels
- Preconception advice for women of childbearing potential, with specialist advice at least 12 weeks prior to stopping contraception (see ➲ Chapters 14 and 15)
- Regular reviews at least every 2 weeks by the diabetes team during pregnancy (see ➲ Chapter 14)
- Good-quality care, with access to diabetes specialists if in hospital (see ➲ Chapter 16)
- A medication review
- Advice on prescription exemption where appropriate
- Discussion/advice on, and facilitation for, access to diabetes technology where appropriate (see ➲ Chapter 6)
- Immunizations, as per national schedule, which may include influenza, pneumococcal, and COVID vaccinations[1]
- Access to condition-specific specialist care for any diabetes-related complications.

An individual diabetes management plan should be discussed and agreed on, which is the result of shared decision-making and takes into consideration a person's cultural background, including personal targets, contact details of the diabetes team, and follow-up plans.

It is vital that a person is seen by the right health care professional, at the right time and in the right place.

Consideration needs to be given to models of integrated care and multidisciplinary teamworking to ensure care standards are met and duplication of care is negated.[2]

For the person with diabetes, it is important to reduce the burden of health care visits and look to promote continuity of care.

In many services, there is a desire to create a 'one-stop shop' model of care delivery where a person can access all health care essentials. An example of this would be the cardio-renal-metabolic clinics, which look to the holistic care of the heart, kidneys, and diabetes in one joined-up review, and multiple long-term conditions clinics.

References

1. UK Health Security Agency (2013, last updated 2020). *Immunisation against infectious disease (The Green Book)*. Available at: ℘ www.gov.uk/government/collections/immunisation-against-infectious-disease-the-green-book
2. Kanumilli N. Delivery of diabetes care in the primary care network structure: a guideline. *Diabetes and Primary Care*. 2021;**23**:37–9. Available at: ℘ https://diabetesonthenet.com/diabetes-primary-care/delivery-diabetes-care-primary-care-network-structure-guideline/

Macrovascular complications of diabetes: prevention and management

Introduction

'Atherosclerotic cardiovascular disease (ASCVD)—defined as coronary heart disease (CHD), cerebrovascular disease, or peripheral arterial disease (PAD), is the leading cause of morbidity and mortality for individuals with diabetes.'[1]

Hypertension and dyslipidaemia are both risk factors for ↑ CVD risk, especially when coexisting with diabetes.

The prevalence of heart failure (HF) in people with diabetes is four times higher than that in the general population, suggesting a pathogenetic role of diabetes.[2]

Other risk factors for CVD and/or HF beyond having diabetes, hypertension, and/or dyslipidaemia include family history in a first-degree relative, smoking, living with obesity, lack of physical activity, and 'poor' diet.

Studies such as STENO-2[3] (undertaken before the use of the newer diabetes therapies which we now know have additional cardiorenal benefit) showed that attainment of glycaemic (HbA1c), blood pressure (BP), and lipid targets can ↑ life expectancy by just under 8 years.

This chapter looks at the optimal management of hypertension and lipids in diabetes, so to reduce CVD and HF risk and, if already established how best to reduce the risk of progression or recurrence.

References

1. ElSayed NA, Aleppo G, Aroda VR, et al.; American Diabetes Association. 7. Diabetes technology: standards of care in diabetes—2023. *Diabetes Care*. 2023;**46**(Suppl 1):S111–27.
2. Rosano GM, Vitale C, Seferovic P. Heart failure in patients with diabetes mellitus. *Cardiac Failure Review*. 2017;**3**(1):52–5.
3. Gæde P, Oellgaard J, Kruuse C, Rossing P, Parving HH, Pedersen O. Beneficial impact of intensified multifactorial intervention on risk of stroke: outcome of 21 years of follow-up in the randomised Steno-2 Study. *Diabetologia*. 2019;**62**(9):1575–80.

Hypertension management in diabetes

Introduction

Hypertension is twice as common in people with diabetes, and the coexistence of diabetes and hypertension significantly ↑ the risk of CHD, left ventricular hypertrophy, HF, and stroke.[1]

Hypertension is also associated with ↑ risk and progression of microvascular complications of diabetes, including nephropathy, retinopathy, and neuropathy (see ➋ Chapter 11).

- BP measurement and individualized target attainment are a vital component of diabetes management, and measurement should be performed at least annually by using validated equipment:
- Correct cuff size
- Gold standard technique:
  - Checking the pulse for any irregular rhythm
  - Measurement in both arms
  - In established hypertension, both sitting and standing BPs to exclude any postural hypotension.

Postural hypotension is associated with autonomic neuropathy (see ➋ Chapter 11).

Blood pressure targets

For a person with diabetes, the National Institute for Health and Care Excellence (NICE) guideline [NG136][2] advises the following preferred BP targets:

- <80 years: <140/90mmHg
- ≥80 years: <150/90mmHg.

For persons with diabetes and chronic kidney disease (CKD), NICE[3] advises the following target BP levels:

- In an adult with CKD and albumin: creatinine ratio (ACR) <70mg/mmol: <140/90mmHg.
- In an adult with CKD and ACR ≥70mg/mmol: <130/80mmHg.

It is important to consider appropriate target BP levels in special circumstances (e.g. those at risk of falls or postural hypotension, those with frailty, reduced life expectancy, or polypharmacy).

Health care professionals (HCPs) also need to be mindful of the risks of lowered BP and consider de-escalation of treatment if a person's systolic BP is <110mmHg.

For adults aged <40 years, consider seeking specialist evaluation for any secondary causes of hypertension.

Diagnosis of hypertension

(See Fig. 10.1)

Lifestyle advice

- Promote healthy eating patterns such as Mediterranean diet or Dietary Approach to Stop Hypertension (DASH).[4]
- Reduce salt intake.
- The DASH eating plan recommends:

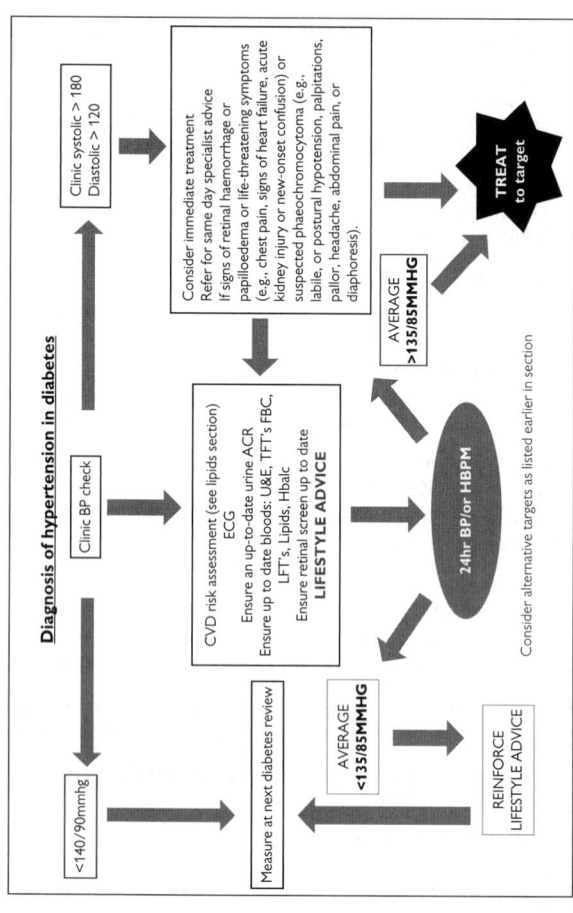

Fig. 10.1 Diagnosis of hypertension in diabetes.

- Standard DASH = 2300mg/day of sodium (6g of salt).
- Lower sodium DASH = 1500mg/day of sodium (3–4g of salt).
- Support individuals to optimize weight if appropriate
- Promote physical activity as appropriate.
- Offer smoking cessation advice where appropriate.
- Provide information about local initiatives that support and promote healthy lifestyles.

Pharmacological treatment of hypertension[2]

Step 1

- Offer an angiotensin-converting enzyme inhibitor (ACEi) or an angiotensin receptor blocker (ARB), in addition to lifestyle advice as above, unless contraindicated.
- Consider an ARB in preference to an ACEi in adults of black African or African Caribbean family origin.
- If an ACEi is not tolerated (e.g. because of cough), offer an ARB.
- Do not combine an ACEi with an ARB to treat hypertension.
- Do not routinely offer an ACEi or ARB if pretreatment serum potassium concentration is >5.0mmol/L and STOP if it rises to ≥6.0mmol/L.
- For women of childbearing potential, see ➲ Chapter 14.

Step 2

- Ensure the person is taking their medications as prescribed.
- Offer a calcium channel blocker or a thiazide-like diuretic, in addition to an ACEi/ARB.
- Indapamide should be used in preference to a conventional thiazide-like diuretic such as bendroflumethiazide or hydrochlorothiazide.

Step 3

- Again, ensure existing medication is being taken as prescribed.
- Use of a calcium channel blocker and a thiazide-like diuretic, in addition to an ACEi/ARB.

Step 4

- Confirm resistant hypertension with ambulatory BP monitoring (ABPM) or home BP monitoring (HBPM); check for postural hypertension, and check medications are taken as prescribed.
- Consider adding low-dose spironolactone if blood potassium concentration is ≤4.5mmol/L, or an α-blocker or a β-blocker if >4.5mmol/L.
- Seek expert advice if BP is uncontrolled on optimal tolerated doses of four drugs.[2]

References

1. Grossman A, Grossman E. Blood pressure control in type 2 diabetic patients. *Cardiovascular Diabetology*. 2017;**16**:3.
2. National Institute for Health and Care Excellence (2019, last updated 2023). *Hypertension in adults: diagnosis and management.* NICE guideline [NG136]. Available at: ℘ www.nice.org.uk/guidance/ng136
3. National Institute for Health and Care Excellence (2021). *Chronic kidney disease: assessment and management.* NICE guideline [NG203]. Available at: ℘ www.nice.org.uk/guidance/ng203

4. Filippou CD, Tsioufis CP, Thomopoulos CG, *et al*. Dietary Approaches to Stop Hypertension (DASH) diet and blood pressure reduction in adults with and without hypertension: a systematic review and meta-analysis of randomized controlled trials. *Advances in Nutrition*. 2020;**11**(5):1150–60.

Further reading

British and Irish Hypertension Society. Educational resources and list of approved home BP monitors. Available at: ℛ https://bihsoc.org

British and Irish Hypertension Society. *Healthy eating diet sheet*. Available at: ℛ https://bihsoc.org/wp-content/uploads/2018/02/Healthy-Eating-Diet-Sheet-Updated-Oct-2017-JH-Final-Feb-2018.pdf

Diabetes UK. *Help with giving up smoking*. Available at: ℛ www.diabetes.org.uk/guide-to-diabetes/life-with-diabetes/help-with-giving-up-smoking

The DASH diet and the Mediterranean diet. Available at: ℛ www.dashdiet.org

Lipid management in diabetes

Lipid management is a key part of the management of diabetes and its complications, including CVD and CKD.

If an individual with diabetes already has these complications, lipid management is a key element of secondary prevention, so statins, along with additional therapies as needed, will be recommended.

In people living with diabetes without the above complications, a primary prevention approach should be taken.

A full non-fasting lipid profile should be recorded, including total cholesterol (TC), high-density lipoprotein cholesterol (HDL-C), and triglycerides.

TC reflects all types of cholesterol in the bloodstream, whereas HDL-C is referred to as 'good' cholesterol, because it works as part of a reverse cholesterol transport system, removing cholesterol from tissues and returning it to the liver for recycling.

The ratio of TC:HDL-C is used to calculate the cardiovascular (CV) risk via tools such as QRISK (see ➲ Further reading, p. 137).

A QRISK score of 10% or more means that lipid-lowering therapies should be considered, along with lifestyle interventions.

In the UK, the Accelerated Access Collaborative (AAC)[1] and NICE[2] guidance both recommend using non-HDL-C as the target value when treating lipids, although low-density lipoprotein cholesterol (LDL-C) values may also be used.

LDL-C is the atherogenic cholesterol which 'furs' up the arteries and is a key component in the development of CVD.

Some national guidelines recommend aiming for a 40% reduction in non-HDL-C, whereas others suggest that an absolute non-HDL-C value of 2.5mmol/L or lower (equivalent to LDL-C of 1.8mmol/L) is preferable.

The European Society of Cardiology (ESC)[3] bases its recommendations for people with established CVD or diabetes on their level of risk—low, moderate, high, or very high—using the risk categories defined in the ESC guideline and this differs from NICE[2] which suggests:

- For primary prevention of CVD:
  - >40% reduction in non-HDL-C.
- For secondary prevention of CVD:
  - LDL-C 2.0mmol/L or lower, or
  - Non-HDL-C 2.6mmol/L or lower.

Triglycerides are made up of fatty acids and glycerol and are an energy source derived from both food and the liver.

Risk factors for raised triglyceride levels include obesity, ↑ sugar or alcohol consumption, and type 2 diabetes (T2D).

There is no guideline-based target for triglycerides, but levels below 1.7mmol/L (or non-fasting levels of 2.3mmol/L) are associated with a reduced risk of CVD.

In type 1 diabetes (T1D), NICE[2] recommends the use of statins for primary prevention in people who:

- Are older than 40 years, or
- Have had T1D for >10 years
- Have established nephropathy, or
- Have other CVD risk factors.

Pharmacological therapies for lipid-lowering

In primary prevention, atorvastatin 20mg is usually recommended, with the potential to add in other therapies, as needed, to get to target.

In secondary prevention, high-intensity statin treatment, such as with atorvastatin 80mg or equivalent, is associated with optimal outcomes.

Ezetimibe is a non-statin lipid-lowering therapy which can effectively reduce LDL-C levels, particularly when taken with a statin. It is usually well tolerated, with few side effects, although gastrointestinal symptoms have been reported. It is prescribed at a dose of 10mg daily.

Bempedoic acid can be prescribed alone (180mg once daily) or in combination with ezetimibe (180/10mg) or with a statin. NICE[4] has recommended bempedoic acid primarily for statin intolerance, but there is evidence to show that it is effective when used with a statin.

Both ezetimibe and bempedoic acid have CV outcome data.

Icosapent ethyl is licensed for secondary prevention of statin-treated or statin-intolerant individuals, or for people with diabetes plus another CV risk factor. NICE[5] recommends icosapent ethyl for secondary prevention to reduce residual CVD risk in people with LDL-C levels of between 1.04mmol/L and 2.6mmol/L and where triglyceride levels remain raised at 1.7mmol/L or above. The dose is 998mg, taken as two capsules, twice daily with food.

Injectable therapies

Inclisiran is a lipid-lowering injection which ↑ the number of LDL-C receptors and hepatic uptake of LDL-C to reduce LDL-C levels by around 50%.

NICE[6] has approved inclisiran for use in secondary prevention, where lipids are not controlled (LDL-C levels of 2.6mmol/L or higher) with other medications or where other drugs are not tolerated.

Side effects are rare and generally limited to injection site tenderness.

PCSK9 inhibitors are also injectable therapies, initiated in secondary care for people who have a history of familial hypercholesterolaemia (FH) or CVD and who are unable to get to target with other lipid-lowering therapies.

Impact of lipid-lowering medications

- Low-intensity statin therapy will produce an LDL-C reduction of 20–30%, medium-intensity statin therapy 31–40%, and high-intensity statin therapy above 40%.
- Ezetimibe, combined with any statin, will potentially result in a greater reduction in non-HDL-C or LDL-C levels than doubling the dose of the statin.
- Bempedoic acid, when combined with ezetimibe, produces an additional LDL-C reduction of ~28%.
- Inclisiran alone or in combination with statins or ezetimibe produces an additional LDL-C reduction of ~50%.
- PCSK9 inhibitors alone or in combination with statins or ezetimibe produce an additional LDL-C reduction of ~50%.

Summary

- In primary prevention, the TC:HDL-C ratio is used to assess risk by using tools such as QRISK, with non-HDL-C or LDL-C values being used for optimizing lipid-lowering therapies.
- It is important to be familiar with contemporaneous local, national, and global guidance on lipid targets and management in diabetes.
- Drugs such as statins, together with lifestyle modifications, can be used along with ezetimibe, bempedoic acid, icosapent ethyl, inclisiran, and PCSK9 inhibitors.

References

1. NHS England/Accelerated Access Collaborative (2022). *Summary of national guidance for lipid management for primary and secondary prevention of CVD.* Available at: ℘ www.england.nhs.uk/aac/wp-content/uploads/sites/50/2020/04/lipid-management-pathway-v7.pdf
2. National Institute for Health and Care Excellence (2023). *Cardiovascular disease: risk assessment and reduction, including lipid modification.* NICE guideline [NG238]. Available at: ℘ www.nice.org.uk/guidance/ng238
3. European Society of Cardiology (2019). *2019 Guidelines on dyslipidaemias (management of).* ESC Clinical Practice Guidelines. Available at: ℘ www.escardio.org/Guidelines/Clinical-Practice-Guidelines/Dyslipidaemias-Management-of
4. National Institute for Health and Care Excellence (2021). *Bempedoic acid with ezetimibe for treating primary hypercholesterolaemia or mixed dyslipidaemia.* Available at: ℘ www.nice.org.uk/guidance/ta694/resources/bempedoic-acid-with-ezetimibe-for-treating-primary-hypercholesterolaemia-or-mixed-dyslipidaemia-pdf-82609440519877
5. National Institute for Health and Care Excellence (2022). *Icosapent ethyl with statin therapy for reducing the risk of cardiovascular events in people with raised triglycerides.* Available at: ℘ www.nice.org.uk/guidance/ta805/resources/icosapent-ethyl-with-statin-therapy-for-reducing-the-risk-of-cardiovascular-events-in-people-with-raised-triglycerides-pdf-82613251568581
6. National Institute for Health and Care Excellence (2021). *Inclisiran for treating primary hypercholesterolaemia or mixed dyslipidaemia.* Available at: ℘ www.nice.org.uk/guidance/ta733

Further reading

Ballantyne CM, Bays H, Catapano AL, et al. Role of bempedoic acid in clinical practice. *Cardiovascular Drugs and Therapy.* 2021;35:853–64.

Cannon CP, Blazing MA, Giugliano RP, et al.; IMPROVE-IT Investigators. Ezetimibe added to statin therapy after acute coronary syndromes. *New England Journal of Medicine.* 2015;372(25):2387–97.

European Society of Cardiology. SCORE2 and SCORE2-OP risk assessment tools. Available at: ℘ www.escardio.org/Education/Practice-Tools/CVD-prevention-toolbox/SCORE-Risk-Charts

Heart UK. Available at: ℘ www.heartuk.org.uk

Nissen SE, et al. (2023). Bempedoic acid for primary prevention of cardiovascular events in statin-intolerant patients. *JAMA.* 2023;330(2):131–40.

Primary Care Cardiovascular Society. Available at: ℘ www.pccsuk.org

QRISK®3 assessment tool. Available at: ℘ www.qrisk.org

Ray KK, Kallend D, Leiter RA, et al.; ORION-11 Investigators. Effect of inclisiran on lipids in primary prevention: the ORION-11 trial. *European Heart Journal.* 2022;43(48):5047–57.

Diabetes, cardiovascular disease, and heart failure

Type 1 diabetes

- In T1D, suboptimal glycaemic levels have been shown to ↑ CV risk 10 times or more, but that optimal glycaemic levels can improve outcomes.
- The Diabetes Control and Complications Trial (DCCT)[1] trial showed that intensive insulin therapy aimed at maintaining HbA1c at near-normal levels resulted in a lower risk of microvascular complications.
- Long-term follow-up showed that the intensive control group continued to have a lower risk of CVD.

Type 2 diabetes

- The United Kingdom Prospective Diabetes Study (UKPDS)[2] in T2D demonstrated that tighter glycaemic and BP control reduced the risk of any diabetes-related end point by 12% and the risk of microvascular disease by 25%.
- There was also a 16% trend towards reducing the risk of myocardial infarction (MI).
- Later analysis of the metformin vs diet control arm showed that the benefit of metformin therapy was maintained across any diabetes-related end point (21%), MI (33%), and all-cause mortality (27%), even if tight control was not maintained in later years—producing the so-called legacy effect.

References

1. Diabetes Control and Complications Trial (DCCT): results of feasibility study. The DCCT Research Group. *Diabetes Care.* 1987;**10**(1):1–19.
2. American Diabetes Association. Implications of the United Kingdom Prospective Diabetes Study. *Diabetes Care.* 2002;**25**(Suppl 1):S28–32.

Cardiovascular risk assessment

Although both T1D and T2D are associated with an ↑ risk of CV complications, CV risk assessment is recommended to quantify an individual's risk, so that treatment can be tailored to optimize the risk:benefit ratio.

The QRISK CV risk assessment tools were developed by using data from the UK General Practice Database. The most recent version of the QRISK tool is QRISK3.

QRISK3 includes a greater number of risk factors, compared with QRISK2 to include:
• Mental illness and medication
• Erectile dysfunction
• CKD stage 3
• Systemic lupus erythematosus
• Migraine.

Existing factors for *QRISK2* include:
• Age
• Gender
• Ethnicity
• Deprivation, based on postcode
• T1D or T2D
• Smoking status
• Atrial fibrillation
• Systolic BP
• TC:HDL-C ratio
• Body mass index
• Rheumatoid arthritis
• CKD stages 4–5.

A score of 10% or more by using QRISK2 or 3 in any individual, with or without diabetes, suggests that medication (e.g. lipid-lowering treatment) is needed, along with lifestyle interventions, to optimize CV risk reduction.

QRISK tools can be accessed at: ℜ www.qrisk.org

Medication that goes beyond glycaemic optimization in type 2 diabetes—sodium–glucose cotransporter 2 inhibitors

Over the years, it has become apparent that some medications used to improve glycaemic levels in T2D have benefits which extend beyond this role. For example, cardiovascular outcomes trials (CVOTs) using sodium–glucose cotransporter 2 (SGLT2) inhibitors have shown that some drugs within this class are associated with improved outcomes for CVD, CKD, and hospitalizations for heart failure (HHF).

The effect of SGLT2 inhibitors on sodium levels and the osmotic effect of raised glucose levels in the urine can help to reduce BP.

SGLT2 inhibition also has a positive impact on the endothelial layer of blood vessels and sodium/hydrogen exchange within the heart and kidney, increasing cardiorenal protection.

The first CVOT to report was the Empagliflozin, Cardiovascular Outcome Event Trial in Type 2 Diabetes Mellitus Patients (EMPA-REG), which involved 7020 people with T2D.

The trial reported a significant reduction in 3-point major adverse cardiovascular events (MACE) in the empagliflozin-treated group vs placebo, and a significant 32% reduction in all-cause mortality, CVD mortality, and HHF.

The reduction in CVD mortality (38%) was driven primarily by a reduction in HHF (35%), as rates of MI and stroke remained unchanged.

The Canagliflozin Cardiovascular Assessment Study (CANVAS) had a larger study population (10,142) and the participants, all of whom had T2D, were a mixture of those with established CVD and those with risk factors for CVD. The results from CANVAS demonstrated a significant reduction in CV events in people with T2D and high CV risk.

The Dapagliflozin and Cardiovascular Outcomes in Type 2 Diabetes trial (DECLARE-TIMI-58) enrolled 17,276 participants with T2D and either established CVD or risk factors for CVD. Although treatment with dapagliflozin in this study group did not impact MACE, it did result in a lower rate of CV death, mainly due to a 27% reduction in HHF.

NICE[1] recommends that SGLT2 inhibitor therapy is considered for people with T2D who have a CVD risk score of 10% or higher to reduce their risk, and for those under the age of 40 years with an elevated lifetime risk of CVD.

NICE also recommends offering SGLT2 inhibition for people with T2D and established CVD or HF.

For more information, see the American Diabetes Association (ADA)/ European Association for the Study of Diabetes (EASD) (2025) consensus statement on the management of hyperglycaemia.[2]

For a summary of trials looking at cardiorenal benefits of SGLT2 inhibitors, see McGuire et al. (2021).[3]

Glucagon-like peptide 1 receptor agonist in type 2 diabetes

The glucagon-like peptide 1 receptor agonists (GLP-1RAs) liraglutide, dulaglutide, and semaglutide have also reported positive CVOTs.

The Liraglutide and Cardiovascular Outcomes (LEADER) trial recruited 9340 individuals who were followed up for a median 3.8 years. Recruits had T2D and were at high risk of a CV event. The primary composite outcome (the first occurrence of death from CV causes, non-fatal MI, or non-fatal stroke) was significantly lower in the liraglutide group and all-cause mortality was also significantly reduced, although CV benefits were seen at around 12–18 months, compared with <3 months with empagliflozin in EMPA-REG.

SUSTAIN-6 used injectable semaglutide in 3297 high-risk individuals, of whom 83% had established CVD, and including CKD. The trial results showed a 26% reduction in the composite primary end point of CV death, non-fatal MI, and non-fatal stroke, with positive changes observed in HbA1c, systolic BP, and weight.

REWIND enrolled 9901 participants to receive dulaglutide or placebo, in addition to their other diabetes medication, for 5.4 years. Just over a third of the trial population had no history of CVD. The primary outcome of MACE occurred in 12% of participants in the treated group and in 13.4% of participants in the placebo group, suggesting a potential benefit. All-cause mortality did not differ between groups.

The ADA and EASD consensus report[2] recommends GLP-1RA therapy for people with T2D, with or at risk of CVD, and for people in whom weight loss is a key consideration.

NB as the book goes to print, we are awaiting the results of the Surpass-CVOT trial for the dual glucose-dependent insulinotropic polypeptide (GIP)/GLP-1RA tirzepatide.

For more information on the role of GLP-1RA therapy in CVD, see Ma et al. (2021).[4]

References

1. National Institute for Health and Care Excellence (2015, last updated 2022). *Type 2 diabetes in adults: management*. NICE guideline [NG28]. Available at: ℘ www.nice.org.uk/guidance/ng28
2. American Diabetes Association Professional Practice Committee; 9. Pharmacologic Approaches to Glycemic Treatment: Standards of Care in Diabetes—2025. *Diabetes Care*. 2025;**48**(Supplement_1):S181–S206. ℘ https://doi.org/10.2337/dc25-S009
3. McGuire DK, Shih WJ, Cosentino F, et al. Association of SGLT2 inhibitors with cardiovascular and kidney outcomes in patients with type 2 diabetes: a meta-analysis. *JAMA Cardiology*. 2021;**6**(2):148–58.
4. Ma X, Liu Z, Ilyas I, et al. (2021). GLP-1 receptor agonists (GLP-1RAs): cardiovascular actions and therapeutic potential. *International Journal of Biological Sciences*. 2021;**17**(8):2050–68.

Heart failure

HF is a condition which carries significant morbidity and mortality. It is also an important comorbidity of T2D, where there is an ↑ risk of developing HF with reduced ejection fraction (HFrEF) and HF with preserved ejection fraction (HFpEF).

In the Framingham study,[1] men with T2D had around double the risk of developing HF, whereas women had closer to five times the level of risk of HF, compared with someone without diabetes.

The role of SGLT2 inhibitors in reducing HHF was seen across populations in all CVOTs, including in people with no previous history of CVD or HF. Based on findings regarding HF in the original CVOTs, further trials were carried out to look at HF outcomes specifically.

The Dapagliflozin and Prevention of Adverse Outcomes in Heart Failure (DAPA-HF) study and the Empagliflozin Outcome Trial in Patients with Chronic Heart Failure and a Reduced Ejection Fraction (EMPEROR-Reduced) both demonstrated significant benefits for SGLT2 inhibitor use in people with HFrEF, with and without diabetes (NB SGLT2 inhibitors are not licensed for use in T1D).

Subsequent trials examined the impact of SGLT2 inhibitors on HFpEF and demonstrated benefits in this group. The Empagliflozin Outcome Trial in Patients with Chronic Heart Failure with Preserved Ejection Fraction (EMPEROR-Preserved) showed that empagliflozin reduced CV death and HHF, and the Dapagliflozin Evaluation to Improve the Lives of Patients with Preserved Ejection Fraction Heart Failure (DELIVER) trial demonstrated that dapagliflozin significantly reduced unplanned HHF, urgent visits for HF, and CV death.

For a summary of the trials using SGLT2 inhibitors in HF, see Talha *et al.* (2023).[2]

The four pillars of heart failure management

For many years, pharmacological management of HF has focused on ACEis (or, more recently, on angiotensin receptor/neprilysin inhibitors), β-blockers, and mineralocorticoid receptor antagonists.

The fourth pillar of HF management in people with HFrEF, with and without diabetes, is now an SGLT2 inhibitor.

In HFpEF, the only drugs which have been shown to have benefit are the SGLT2 inhibitors dapagliflozin and empagliflozin.

For ESC guidelines on HF, see European Society of Cardiology (2021).[3]

For NICE guidelines on HF, see National Institute for Health and Care Excellence (2018).[4]

References

1. Framingham Heart Study. Ongoing research Available at: ℘ www.framinghamheartstudy.org/
2. Talha KM, Anker SD, Butler J. SGLT-2 inhibitors in heart failure: a review of current evidence. *International Journal of Heart Failure.* 2023;**5**(2):82–90.
3. European Society of Cardiology (2021). *2021 ESC Guidelines for the diagnosis and treatment of acute and chronic heart failure. ESC Clinical Practice Guidelines.* Available at: ℘ www.escardio.org/ Guidelines/Clinical-Practice-Guidelines/Acute-and-Chronic-Heart-Failure
4. National Institute for Health and Care Excellence (2018). *Chronic heart failure in adults: diagnosis and management.* NICE guideline [NG106]. Available at: ℘ www.nice.org.uk/guidance/ng106

Summary

- Studies have shown that both T1D and T2D confer CV risk and that optimizing blood glucose levels, along with BP and lipid management, may reduce that risk.
- To quantify an individual's level of risk, tools such as QRISK can be used, with relevant interventions recommended in people with scores of 10% or higher.
- A combination of lifestyle interventions, along with pharmacological treatments (SGLT2 inhibitors, GLP-1RAs, ACEis, and statins), can then be tailored to optimize benefits.
- People with T2D should be offered an explanation as to the cardiorenal benefits of drugs such as SGLT2 inhibitors and GLP-1RAs beyond glycaemic control, along with information about possible side effects, as shared decision-making is essential.
- NICE recommends the use of SGLT2 inhibitors in people with, or at risk of, CVD, and the ADA/EASD consensus report takes a holistic approach to diabetes care by recognizing the cardioprotective benefits of SGLT2 inhibitors and GLP-1RAs.
- Preventing or slowing down the impact of costly complications, such as CV events, diabetic kidney disease, and HF, requires proactive use of these drugs.

Case study

Mrs Jones is a 68-year-old lady with T2D for the last 7 years.
- HbA1c 48mmol/mol
- BP 150/90mmHg
- Lipid profile: TC 4.2mmol/L, non-HDL-C 3.0mmol/L, HDL-C 1.0mmol/L, LDL-C 2.9mmol/L
- Estimated glomerular filtration rate (eGFR) 90
- Urine microalbumin 3.6mmol/L
- Body mass index (BMI) 34kg/m²
- Smokes 10 cigarettes a day
- Current medications are: metformin 1g twice daily, ramipril 5mg daily

Question

What advice, support, and management would you give Mrs Jones to reduce her risk of CV complications?

Answers

1. Explain the association of diabetes with hypertension and suboptimal lipids.
2. Explain the association of diabetes, suboptimal lipids, hypertension, smoking, and higher BMI with cardiovascular risk
3. Offer lifestyle support and signposting to resources, including those for:
   a. Smoking cessation
   b. Support with weight loss
   c. Diabetes education
   d. Dietary interventions to support CV risk reduction
   e. Physical activity interventions as appropriate.
4. Manage hypertension:
   a. Check if taking ramipril as prescribed.
   b. Optimise ramipril dose to 10mg daily and then add further BP-lowering medications as required and with consent.
   c. Follow-up review of BP values, including, if possible, home monitoring values.
5. Optimize lipid levels:
   a. Undertake QRISK assessment (for Mrs Jones, this is >30%).
   b. Start atorvastatin 20mg with consent and as per summary of product characteristics (SMPC).
   c. Ongoing review of the effectiveness of statin, with repeat lipid profiles at least annually, intensifying lipid-lowering therapy as per lipid profile values.
6. Add in SGLT2 inhibitor therapy, with evidence of benefit in those at high risk of CVD, with consent and as per SMPC, with appropriate advice on possible side effects and sick day guidance (see ➜ Chapter 2).

Microvascular complications of diabetes: prevention and management

Introduction

Microvascular complications of diabetes are long-term complications that affect small blood vessels. These typically include retinopathy, nephropathy, and neuropathy.

Microvascular complications usually develop over several years but can manifest even at diagnosis, particularly in people with type 2 diabetes (T2D) who may have had the condition for a number of years before diagnosis.

The 'DISCOVER'[1] observational study programme from 2014 to 2019 reported that the global crude prevalence of microvascular complications in people with T2D was 18.8%.

There is a strong correlation between vascular-related complications of diabetes. For example, diabetic retinopathy is strongly associated with the risk of developing diabetic kidney disease which is a strong predictor of stroke and cardiovascular disease (CVD).

Multiple complications are associated with doubling of cardiovascular (CV) risk and CV mortality.[2]

Multifactorial intervention, including optimal management of hyperglycaemia, blood pressure, lipids, and smoking cessation, is the cornerstone of good management to improve microvascular health (see also ➔ Chapters 7 and 10).

This chapter will look at specific potential microvascular complications in diabetes to support prevention, detection, and optimal management of these conditions.

References

1. Kosiborod M, Gomes MB, Nicolucci A, *et al*. Vascular complications in patients with type 2 diabetes: Prevalence and associated factors in 38 countries (the DISCOVER study program). *Cardiovascular Diabetology*. 2018;**17**(1):150. Available at: ⅏ https://doi.org/10.1186/s12 933-018-0787-8

2. Crasto W, Patel V, Davies MJ, Khunti K. (2021) Prevention of microvascular complications of diabetes, endocrinology and metabolism. *Clinics of North America*. 2021;**50**(3):431–55. Available at: ⅏ https://doi.org/10.1016/j.ecl.2021.05.005

Renal complications in diabetes: assessment, risk reduction, and management

Background

This section will cover chronic kidney disease (CKD) in diabetes and, briefly, acute kidney injury (AKI).

CKD affects 20–40% of people with diabetes and is defined by persistent elevation of urinary albumin excretion (albuminuria), low estimated glomerular filtration rate (eGFR), or other manifestations of kidney damage.[1]

Almost one in five people with diabetes will need treatment for kidney disease during their lifetime.[2]

CKD can progress to end-stage renal disease (ESRD) requiring dialysis or kidney transplantation, and is the leading cause of ESRD. In addition, the presence of CKD is associated with significantly elevated CV risk.[3]

Function of the kidneys

- Regulation of acid–base balance.
- Regulation of fluid balance.
- Maintenance of electrolyte balance.
- Removal of toxins and waste products from the body.
- Role in blood pressure regulation.
- Production of the hormone erythropoietin.
- Activation of vitamin D.

Risk factors for chronic kidney disease

- ↑ age.
- Diabetes.
- Hypertension.
- CVD.
- Nephrotoxic drugs.
- Smoking.
- Multisystem disease.
- African, African-Caribbean, or Asian family origin.
- Positive family history of renal disease.
- Previous history of AKI.

NB not all cases of CKD in people with diabetes are caused by diabetes. It is important to recognize other causes (autoimmune disease, renal artery stenosis, obstruction, malignancy, and myeloma) that need to be investigated and treated differently.

Risk reduction of chronic kidney disease in diabetes

- Optimization of blood pressure (see ➋ Chapter 10).
- Early screening for T2D.
- Optimization of glucose levels (see ➋ Chapter 7).
- Smoking cessation where appropriate.
- Promotion of lifestyle for a healthy weight (see ➋ Chapter 4).
- Review of potentially nephrotoxic medications, including non-steroidal anti-inflammatory drugs (NSAIDs).

Screening for chronic kidney disease in diabetes

Estimated glomerular filtration rate (eGFR)

Glomerular filtration rate describes the flow rate of filtered fluid through the kidney. The National Institute for Health and Care Excellence (NICE) advises that whenever a request for serum creatinine measurement is made, clinical laboratories should report an estimate of eGFRcreatinine by using a prediction equation, in addition to reporting the serum creatinine result.[4] This measurement should be taken at least annually when screening people with diabetes.

NB eGFRcreatinine may be less reliable in certain situations (e.g. AKI, pregnancy, oedematous states, muscle wasting disorders, and in adults who are malnourished, have higher muscle mass, or use protein supplements, or those who have had an amputation) and has not been well validated in certain ethnic groups (e.g. black, Asian, and other minority ethnic groups) with CKD living in the UK.[4]

NB People should be advised not to eat any meat in the 12 hours before having a blood test for eGFRcreatinine.

For further information, see NICE guideline [NG203].[4]

Urine albumin:creatinine ratio

This is a measurement of urine albumin. Normally, the kidneys filter albumin, so if albumin is found in the urine, this is a marker of kidney disease. This measurement should be undertaken at least annually for screening in people with diabetes. A raised urine albumin:creatinine ratio (ACR) is the earliest indicator of kidney damage and can be raised even if the eGFR is normal.

A positive result is one where the urine microalbumin content is >3mg/mmol.

The sample can be taken from an 'on-the-spot' urine collection, but if found to be >3mg/mmol and <70mg/mmol, then a second early-morning sample is required to confirm the first diagnosis. If the initial result is >70mg/mmol, a repeat sample is not required.

NB relevant to exclude any haematuria or overt proteinuria by dipstick testing ahead of sending a urine sample to the laboratory for ACR measurement.

NB overt proteinuria may be due to other causes (e.g. urinary tract infection).

For further information, see NICE guideline [NG203].[4]

Diagnosis and classification of chronic kidney disease in diabetes

CKD is usually a clinical diagnosis made based on the presence of albuminuria and/or reduced eGFR in the absence of signs or symptoms of other primary causes of kidney damage (see Fig. 11.1).[1] Often the presentation is associated with long-standing duration of diabetes, retinopathy, albuminuria, and gradually progressive loss of eGFR but may present at onset in T2D, especially if a late diagnosis and other risk factors, such as hypertension, have been present.

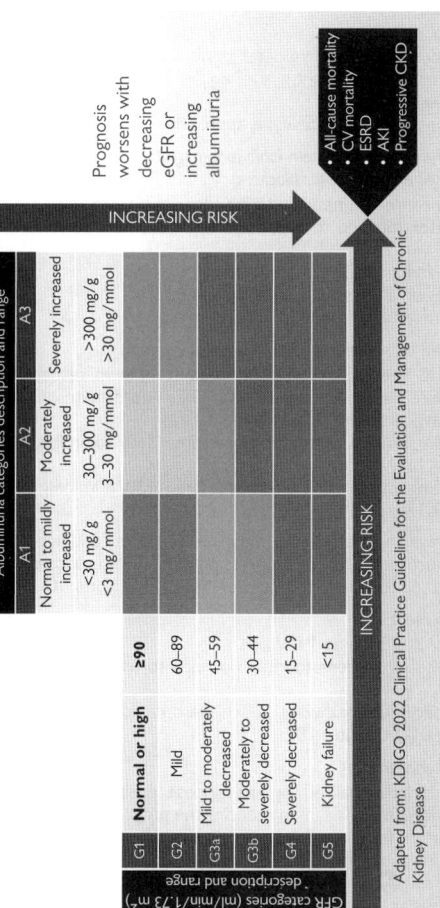

Measures of kidney function and markers of kidney damage are required to identify those who are at increased risk of progression

GFR categories (ml/min/1.73 m²) description and range			Albuminuria categories description and range		
			A1	A2	A3
			Normal to mildly increased	Moderately increased	Severely increased
			<30 mg/g <3 mg/mmol	30–300 mg/g 3–30 mg/mmol	>300 mg/g >30 mg/mmol
G1	Normal or high	≥90			
G2	Mild	60–89			
G3a	Mild to moderately decreased	45–59			
G3b	Moderately to severely decreased	30–44			
G4	Severely decreased	15–29			
G5	Kidney failure	<15			

INCREASING RISK

INCREASING RISK

Prognosis worsens with decreasing eGFR or increasing albuminuria

- All-cause mortality
- CV mortality
- ESRD
- AKI
- Progressive CKD

Adapted from: KDIGO 2022 Clinical Practice Guideline for the Evaluation and Management of Chronic Kidney Disease

Fig. 11.1 Classification of chronic kidney disease based on urine ACR and eGFR values.

Kidney Disease: Improving Global Outcomes (KDIGO) Diabetes Work Group. KDIGO 2024 clinical practice guideline for the evaluation and management of chronic kidney disease. *Kidney International.* 2024;**105**(Suppl 4S):S117–314. Available at: ℔ https://kdigo.org/wp-content/uploads/2024/03/KDIGO-2024-CKD-Guideline.pdf

Management of chronic kidney disease in diabetes

Optimal management of CKD is important in reducing its progression and morbidity.

Lifestyle advice
- Education.
- Smoking cessation if appropriate.
- Support for healthy weight.
- Reduced salt intake.
- Promotion of physical activity as appropriate.

Use of renin–angiotensin system inhibitors (angiotensin-converting enzyme inhibitors/angiotensin receptor blockers)
NICE guidance[4] recommends offering a low-cost renin–angiotensin system (RAS) inhibitor (titrated to the maximum tolerated dose) to people with CKD and:
- Diabetes and an ACR of ≥3mg/mmol
- Hypertension and an ACR of ≥30mg/mmol
- An ACR of ≥70mg/mmol.

Blood pressure management
National[4] and international guidance[1] may vary with respect to optimal blood pressure targets for people with CKD and diabetes. Current NICE guidance[4] advocates for:
- ACR <70mg/mmol: clinic blood pressure <140/90mmHg (home readings <135/85mmHg)
- ACR >70mg/mmol: clinic blood pressure <130/80mmHg (home readings <125/75mmHg).

NB it is always important to individualize BP targets and agents according to age, comorbidities, risk of progression of CKD, presence or absence of retinopathy, and tolerance to treatment (see ➜ Chapter 10).

Lipid management
People with CKD have an ↑ CV risk.[3]
   This is a cohort where there is no need to use QRISK, as the risk is defined.
   Lipid management pathways to achieve optimal lipid profiles should be followed (see ➜ Chapter 10).

Glycaemic management
Attainment of individualised/optimal glucose levels, including HbA1c and/or time in range, is significant in reducing the progression of CKD.[5]
   It is important to remember that as a person's renal function declines:
- Some medications for T2D may need to be dose-adjusted or stopped (see ➜ Chapter 2). Insulin may need to be initiated as other medications are reduced or stopped.
- There is an ↑ risk of hypoglycaemia, and thus glycaemic targets may need to be individualized for persons using a sulfonylurea and/or insulin (see ➜ Chapters 7 and 12).

Renal effects of sodium–glucose cotransporter 2 inhibitors

The American Diabetes Association (ADA)[6] advises that sodium–glucose cotransporter 2 (SGLT2) inhibitors, via mechanisms independent of glycaemia, reduce:

- Renal tubular glucose reabsorption
- Weight
- Systolic blood pressure
- Intraglomerular pressure
- Albuminuria, and
- Slow GFR loss.

Key randomized controlled trials in support of the use of SGLT2 inhibitors in people with diabetes and CKD reflect some of the secondary end point outcomes of the cardiovascular outcomes trials (CVOTs) described in ➋ Chapter 10. Renal-specific trials include CREDENCE (canagliflozin),[7] DAPA-CKD (dapagliflozin),[8] and EMPA-KIDNEY (empagliflozin).[9]

Both national and international guidance now support the early use of SGLT2 inhibitors independent of the need for glucose-lowering effect, so to enable potential cardiorenal benefits (see ➋ Chapters 2 and 10).

Glucose-lowering efficacy of SGLT2 inhibitor therapy is reduced if the eGFR is persistently <45mL/min/1.73m², and almost non-existent if <30mL/min/1.73m². It remains important to use an SGLT2 inhibitor as licensed for cardiorenal protection, but if a reduction in glycaemia is also required, then another agent such as a glucagon-like peptide 1 receptor agonist (GLP-1RA) may need to be introduced.

Please refer to individual summary of product characteristics (SMPCs) for each SGLT2 inhibitor for contemporaneous indications of use.

NB at the time of writing, results of the FLOW Trial[9] comparing the effects of semaglutide 1mg (a GLP-1RA) with placebo as an adjunct to standard of care on kidney outcomes for the prevention of progression of renal impairment and risk of renal and CV mortality had just been published. These showed that semaglutide reduced the risk of clinically important kidney outcomes and death from CV causes in people with T2D and CKD. Further trial results are awaited for other classes of incretin therapy.

Other considerations

Non-steroidal mineralocorticoid receptor antagonists

National[4] and international guidance[1,11] suggests consideration of non-steroidal mineralocorticoid receptor antagonists with proven kidney or CV benefit for people with T2D, an eGFR >25mL/min/1.73m², normal serum potassium concentration, and albuminuria >3mg/mmol, in addition to the maximum tolerated dose of a RAS inhibitor.

This is based on data from the Finerenone in Reducing Kidney Failure and Disease Progression in Diabetic Kidney Disease (FIDELIO-DKD)[12] and Finerenone in Reducing Cardiovascular Mortality and Morbidity in Diabetic Kidney Disease (FIGARO-DKD) trials,[13] which demonstrated that finerenone, on top of angiotensin-converting enzyme inhibitor (ACEi) or angiotensin receptor blocker (ARB) treatment, slows progressive loss of eGFR and ↓ the risk of CV events in people with T2D and albuminuria.

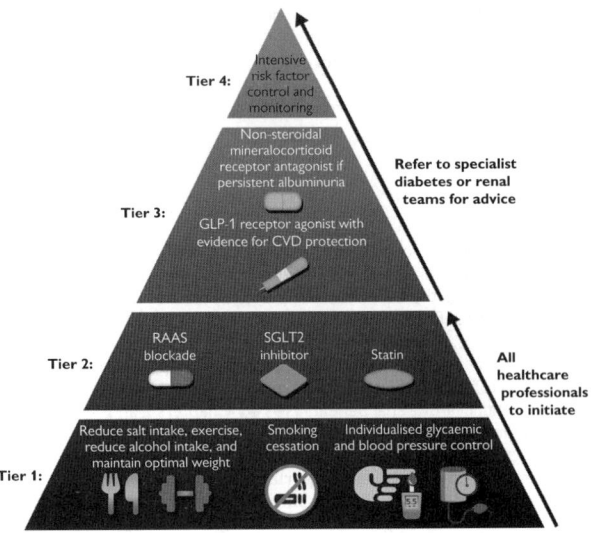

Fig. 11.2 Four-tier approach to managing chronic kidney disease in diabetes.
Reference Dasgupta I, Zac-Varghese S, Chaudhry K, *et al*. Current management of chronic kidney disease in type-2 diabetes—A tiered approach: An overview of the joint Association of British Clinical Diabetologists and UK Kidney Association (ABCD-UKKA) guidelines. *Diabet Med*. 2024;00:e15450. doi:10.1111/dme.15450

Antiplatelet therapy

Antiplatelet medication may be offered to persons with CKD for primary prevention of CVD based on specialist advice.

Other considerations

- Screening for possible anaemia.
- For people with eGFR <30mL/min/1.73m², it is relevant to check vitamin D levels and bone profile.

Kidney Failure Risk Equation

By using a person's urine ACR, sex, age, and eGFR, the Kidney Failure Risk Equation (KFRE) provides the 2- and 5-year probability of treated kidney failure for a potential person with CKD stages 3a–5 (available at: 🔗 https://kidneyfailurerisk.co.uk/).

When to refer to specialist renal care

It is relevant to be aware of local referral pathways.
    NICE guidance[4] is to consider referral in the following circumstances:
- A 5-year risk of needing renal replacement therapy of >5% (measured by using the 4-variable KFRE)

- ACR of 70mg/mmol or greater, unless known to be caused by diabetes and already appropriately treated
- ACR of >30mg/mmol, together with haematuria
- Sustained ↓ in eGFR of 25% or greater and a change in eGFR category within 12 months
- Sustained ↓ in eGFR of 15mL/min/1.73m² or greater per year
- Hypertension that remains poorly controlled (above the person's individual target) despite the use of at least four antihypertensive medicines at therapeutic doses
- Known or suspected rare or genetic causes of CKD
- Suspected renal artery stenosis.

Case study

Mrs Ahmad is a 57-year-old lady with T2D for 8 years:
- Body mass index 32.4kg/m²
- Non-smoker
- HbA1c 51mmol/mol
- Total cholesterol 4.2mmol/L, triglycerides 2.0, serum non-high-density lipoprotein (HDL) cholesterol 2.8
- Urine ACR >3 on two occasions (3.2 and 3.6mmol/L)
- eGFR 89mL/min/1.73m²
- Blood pressure 130/80mmHg
- Current medications: metformin 1g twice daily, ramipril 2.5mg once daily.

Question

How would you look to provide support and optimization of Mrs Ahmad's care to reduce the risk of renal progression?

Answers

1. Education on the association between diabetes and CKD, and how to reduce the risk of progression.
2. Offer lifestyle advice and support to achieve a healthy weight.
3. Optimize the dose of ramipril, aiming to titrate to 10mg daily, provided blood pressure readings do not lower to an unacceptable level.
4. Look to start a statin, with consent (no need to perform a QRISK assessment).
5. Look to introduce an SGLT2 inhibitor with renal benefit, as per SMPC, with appropriate advice given on possible side effects and sick day guidance (see ➲ Chapter 2).
6. Agree timely follow-up for repeat bloods and ongoing review.

Acute kidney injury

AKI, previously known as acute renal failure (ARF), is diagnosed with sustained ↑ in serum creatinine level of 50% or greater over a short period of time, which is also reflected as rapid ↓ in eGFR. The new terminology highlights that AKI presents as a spectrum, from mild kidney injury to severe kidney failure.[14] Diabetes is a distinct risk factor for AKI.

Incidence

The incidence of AKI in people with diabetes is 4.7 times higher, compared with the non-diabetic population.[15] Studies have also shown that people with T2D show a steeper eGFR decline prior to AKI, compared with individuals without diabetes.

Causes

AKI is a clinical syndrome that is caused by a wide range of disorders. Three syndromes can be used to help classify AKI:

- Prerenal (most common)—due to reduced blood flow in the kidneys and/or hypotension, leading to a fall in eGFR; usually reversible with appropriate early treatment[15]
- Intrarenal—due to structural damage to the kidney; it may result from persistent prerenal or post-renal causes, which may lead to renal cell damage
- Post-renal (least common)—due to acute obstruction of urine flow within the renal tract, resulting in ↑ intratubular pressure and ↓ eGFR.

Increased risk of acute kidney injury in diabetes See Fig 11.3

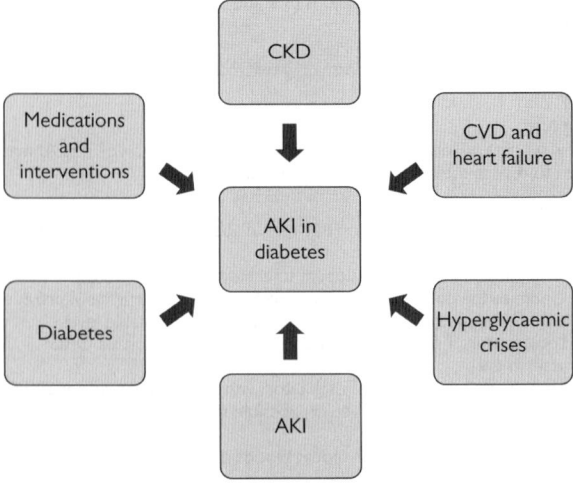

Fig. 11.3 Multiple factors increasing the risk of AKI in people with diabetes.

Identification

There are several criteria to identify AKI.

The most used tool is Kidney Disease: Improving Global Outcomes (KDIGO),[16] which identifies AKI as the presence of any of the following:

- ↑ serum creatinine level by 0.3mg/dL or more (26.5μmol/L or more) within 48 hours

- ↑ serum creatinine level to 1.5 times or more than the baseline of the previous 7 days
- Urine output of <0.5mL/kg/hour for at least 6 hours.

Monitor serum creatinine level regularly in all adults with, or at risk of, AKI. Daily monitoring is required for patients in hospital.

Diabetes medication management in acute kidney injury

Metformin

There is strong evidence suggesting the benefits of metformin in reducing the risk of AKI by preserving kidney function. It can reduce oxidative stress, which will help to protect renal tubular cells.[17] However, metformin can accumulate in AKI, leading to lactic acidosis. Hence, care should be taken when starting metformin in people at risk of AKI. Also metformin must be stopped if AKI is diagnosed, but it can be safely restarted once renal function returns to normal.

Sulfonylureas

Sulfonylureas must be stopped in AKI due to ↑ risk of hypoglycaemia related to reduced renal clearance.

Dipeptidyl peptidase type 4 inhibitors

These drugs must generally be stopped in AKI, as they will accumulate due to reduced renal clearance. The only drug which can be used safely is linagliptin, as it requires minimal renal clearance. However, there is lack of evidence to suggest that linagliptin is effective in managing hyperglycaemia in people with AKI.

Sodium–glucose cotransporter 2 inhibitors

These drugs can protect the kidney by reducing hyperfiltration, decreasing inflammation, and increasing tubular cell survival. Studies have shown that SGLT2 inhibitors can reduce the risk of AKI by 23% in people with or without diabetes. A reduced baseline eGFR should be considered a risk of AKI when people with diabetes are being started on this class of drugs. These drugs must be paused short term in people with AKI to prevent adverse effects (see ➡ Chapter 2) until renal function has recovered.

Insulin

This is the safest therapy for management of hyperglycaemia in people with AKI. However, there is an ↑ risk of hypoglycaemia due to reduced clearance of insulin. Hence, it is important to reduce insulin doses if renal function starts to deteriorate. Increasing the frequency of glucose monitoring is important, and the use of shorter-acting insulins may be preferable.

General management of acute kidney injury

Factors such as stage of AKI, age, comorbidities, risk of complications, and social situation must be taken into consideration when assessing whether to arrange hospital admission, liaison with a specialist, or ongoing management in primary care.

Arrange urgent hospital admission if

- Likely stage 3 AKI
- An underlying cause requiring urgent hospital management such as suspected urinary tract obstruction and/or upper urinary tract infection
- No identifiable cause for AKI
- Risk of urinary tract obstruction
- Sepsis
- Evidence of hypovolaemia and need for intravenous fluid replacement
- Deterioration in clinical condition or need for ↑ frequency of observation which is not possible in the primary care setting
- A complication of AKI that requires urgent hospital admission such as pulmonary oedema, uraemic encephalopathy, or severe hyperkalaemia.

Liaise with a nephrologist as soon as possible if

- Stage 4 or 5 CKD
- A possible diagnosis that may need specialist treatment such as tubulointerstitial nephritis, glomerulonephritis, systemic vasculitis, or myeloma
- An inadequate response to treatment in primary care
- A history of renal transplant.

STOP AKI is a simple care bundle that can be used to manage AKI effectively (see Box 11.1).[18]

Prevention

- Be cautious when using volume-depleting drugs (SGLT2 inhibitors and diuretics), drugs affecting perfusion (ACEis/ARBs/NSAIDs), or iodine-containing contrast for radiological investigations in people with diabetes.
- People must be educated on understanding which drugs to continue, when to omit them, and when to carefully restart them (e.g. in cases of any dehydrating illness).
- People who have their medications in a dosette box should be advised to seek medical advice if unwell, so that guidance on which tablet(s) to omit can be explained.
- Regular monitoring by primary care teams on how to reduce the risk of developing AKI, optimizing diabetes and other medication doses, and regular monitoring of renal function are important.[19]

Box 11.1 STOP AKI care bundle

Sepsis—urgent sepsis screen to be completed and initiate local care bundle

Toxins—identify and stop

Optimize volume status and blood pressure—consider withholding diuretics and hypertensive medications

Prevent harm—identify and treat reversible causes such as urinary tract obstruction, hyperkalaemia, and acidosis

Post-acute kidney injury care
- Optimize medicine management.
- Renal function must be checked 3 months after an episode of AKI for new-onset, worsening, or pre-existing CKD. Earlier monitoring is needed if serum creatinine level has not returned to pre-AKI baseline.
- Communicate kidney health and AKI risk with people with diabetes and their carers. Sick day guidance must be discussed, with advice regarding cessation of medicines during specific acute illnesses (see ➲ chapter 17).
- Embed post-AKI care planning into routine practice by establishing a primary care practice protocol.

References

1. ElSayed NA, Aleppo G, Aroda VR, *et al.*; American Diabetes Association. 11. Chronic kidney disease and risk management: standards of care in diabetes—2023. *Diabetes Care.* 2023;**46**(Suppl 1):S191–202. Available at: ℬ https://doi.org/10.2337/dc23-S011
2. Diabetes UK (2019). *Us, diabetes and a lot of facts and stats.* Available at: ℬ www.diabetes.org.uk/resources-s3/2019-11/facts-stats-update-oct-2019.pdf
3. Morales, J, Handelsman, Y. Cardiovascular outcomes in patients with diabetes and kidney disease: *JACC* Review Topic of the Week. *Journal of American College of Cardiology.* 2023;**82**(2):161–70. Available at: ℬ https://doi.org/10.1016/j.jacc.2023.04.052
4. National Institute for Health and Care Excellence (2021). *Chronic kidney disease: assessment and management.* NICE guideline [NG203]. Available at: ℬ www.nice.org.uk/guidance/ng203
5. King P, Peacock I, Donnelly R. The UK prospective diabetes study (UKPDS): clinical and therapeutic implications for type 2 diabetes. *British Journal of Clinical Pharmacology.* 1999;**48**(5):643–8.
6. American Diabetes Association Primary Care Advisory Group; Introduction: Standards of Care in Diabetes—2024 Abridged for Primary Care Professionals. *Clin Diabetes* 15 April 2024;**42**(2):181. ℬ https://doi.org/10.2337/cd24-aint
7. Perkovic V, Jardine MJ, Neal B, *et al.*; CREDENCE Trial Investigators. Canagliflozin and Renal Outcomes in Type 2 Diabetes and Nephropathy. *New England Journal of Medicine.* 2019;**380**(24):2295–306.
8. Heerspink HJL, Stefánsson BV, Correa-Rotter R, *et al.*; DAPA-CKD Trial Committees and Investigators. Dapagliflozin in Patients with Chronic Kidney Disease. *New England Journal of Medicine.* 2020;**383**(15):1436–46.
9. The EMPA-KIDNEY Collaborative Group; Herrington WG, Staplin N, Wanner C, *et al.* Empagliflozin in Patients with Chronic Kidney Disease. *New England Journal of Medicine.* 2023;**388**(2):117–27.
10. Perkovic V, Tuttle KR, Rossing P, *et al.*; FLOW Trial Committees and Investigators. Effects of semaglutide on chronic kidney disease in patients with type 2 diabetes. *New England Journal of Medicine.* 2024;**391**(2):109–21.
11. Kidney Disease: Improving Global Outcomes (KDIGO) Diabetes Work Group. KDIGO 2024 clinical practice guideline for the evaluation and management of chronic kidney disease. *Kidney International.* 2024;**105**(Suppl 4S):S117–314. Available at: ℬ https://kdigo.org/wp-content/uploads/2024/03/KDIGO-2024-CKD-Guideline.pdf
12. Filippatos G, Anker SD, Agarwal R, *et al.*; FIDELIO-DKD Investigators. Finerenone and cardiovascular outcomes in patients with chronic kidney disease and type 2 diabetes. *Circulation.* 2021;**143**:540–52.
13. Pitt B, Filippatos G, Agarwal R, *et al.*; FIGARO-DKD Investigators. Cardiovascular events with finerenone in kidney disease and type 2 diabetes. *New England Journal of Medicine.* 2021;**385**:2252–63.
14. Kidney Disease: Improving Global Outcomes (KDIGO) Acute Kidney Injury Work Group. KDIGO clinical practice guideline for acute kidney injury. *Kidney International Supplements.* 2012;**2**:1–138.
15. BMJ Best Practice (2024). *Acute kidney injury.* Available at: ℬ https://bestpractice.bmj.com/topics/en-gb/3000117/pdf/3000117/Acute%20kidney%20injury.pdf
16. Pereira M, Rodrigues N, Godinho I, *et al.* Acute kidney injury in patients with severe sepsis or septic shock: a comparison between the 'Risk, Injury, Failure, Loss of kidney function, End-stage

kidney disease' (RIFLE), Acute Kidney Injury Network (AKIN) and Kidney Disease: Improving Global Outcomes (KDIGO) classifications. *Clinical Kidney Journal*. 2017;**10**(3):332–40.

17. Gui Y, Palanza Z, Fu H, Zhou D. Acute kidney injury in diabetes mellitus: epidemiology, diagnostic and therapeutic concepts. *FASEB Journal*. 2023;**37**:e22884. Available at: ℘ https://faseb.onlinelibrary.wiley.com/doi/epdf/10.1096/fj.202201340RR

18. Royal College of Physicians (2015). *Acute care toolkit 12: acute kidney injury and intravenous fluid therapy*. Available at: ℘ www.rcplondon.ac.uk/guidelines-policy/acute-care-toolkit-12-acute-kidney-injury-and-intravenous-fluid-therapy

19   Geeky Medics (2021, last updated 2024). *Acute kidney injury (AKI)*. Available at: ℘ https://geekymedics.com/acute-kidney-injury-aki

Further reading

Diabetes UK. *Diabetes: keeping your kidneys healthy*. [Information prescriptions for health care professionals] Available at: ℘ https://www.diabetes.org.uk/for-professionals/supporting-your-patients/information-prescriptions/information-prescriptions-qa

Diabetes UK. *Diabetes and kidney disease*. [Information prescriptions for health care professionals] Available at: ℘ https://www.diabetes.org.uk/for-professionals/supporting-your-patients/information-prescriptions/information-prescriptions-qa

National Kidney Foundation. Available at: ℘ www.kidney.org/

Think Kidneys (2016). *When or if to re-start ACEI, ARB, diuretics and other antihypertensive drugs after an episode of acute kidney injury*. Available at: ℘ www.thinkkidneys.nhs.uk/aki/wp-content/uploads/sites/2/2016/02/When-to-restart-drugs-stopped-during-AKI-final.pdf

Think Kidneys (2018). *'Sick day' guidance in patients at risk of acute kidney injury: a position statement from the Think Kidneys Board*. Available at: ℘ www.thinkkidneys.nhs.uk/aki/wp-content/uploads/sites/2/2018/01/Think-Kidneys-Sick-Day-Guidance-2018.pdf

The diabetic foot

Background

Diabetes is the leading cause of lower limb amputation in the UK. People with diabetes are 23 times more likely to have a leg, foot or toe amputation than someone without diabetes.[1] Of all the lower extremity amputations in persons with diabetes, 85% are preceded by a foot ulcer.[2] It is estimated that the lifetime risk of developing a diabetic foot ulcer is between 19–34%. The early detection of diabetic foot ulcers combined with appropriate treatment is known to reduce the risk of amputation.

Not all people with diabetes are at risk of developing a foot ulcer. It is often the combination of the loss of protective sensation known as neuropathy, infection and peripheral arterial disease which can lead to an increased risk of lower limb amputation.[3] Therefore, it is imperative that foot ulcer prevention and education is a priority for all health care professionals involved in the care of people with diabetes.

The 'stairway to an amputation' depicts the most common compounding steps leading to limb loss in those with diabetes (see Fig. 11.4).[3]

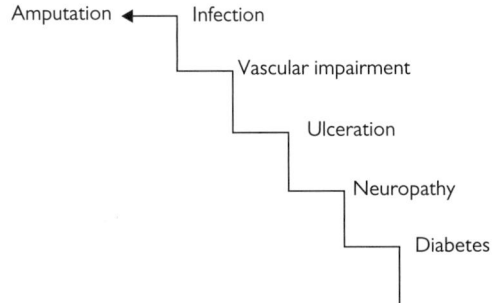

Fig. 11.4 The stairway to amputation.

Diabetes foot assessments

The National Institute for Health and Care Excellence (NICE) diabetic foot guidance[4] stipulates that all people with diabetes should have a foot examination at the following times:
- Upon diagnosis and then at regular intervals depending on their risk factors.
- If any foot problems develop.
- Upon admission to hospital or if there is any change in status during their inpatient stay.

Foot assessment check list and questions to ask people with diabetes:
- Remove shoes, socks and any dressings
- Is the skin intact?
- Check in between the toes

- Are there any signs of necrosis?
- Is there any callus present?
- Is the shape of the foot normal?
- Does the foot feel red hot or swollen?
- Ask the person if they can feel their feet
- Does the person have a history of foot ulceration?
- Are the foot pulses palpable?
- Does the person complain of any pain, numbness, tingling sensations
- Can the person safely perform their own foot care and if not are they known to their local podiatry service?

Both NICE and the international working group for the diabetic foot (IWGDF)[5] recommend that individuals are assessed using a clear risk stratification system. It is important to know what action to take depending on the person's risk level and for HCPs to be familiar with local referral pathways and protocols especially in respect of an active foot ulcer. Table 11.1 below describes the risk levels and the corresponding action that must be taken.

Table 11.1 Risk levels and corresponding actions based on the findings of the diabetes foot examination

Risk	Action
Low:	
No risk factors present except callus alone.	Provide foot care education and the contact details of local podiatry services
	Screen once per year
Moderate:	
Deformity, neuropathy or peripheral arterial disease (PAD)	Provide foot care education.
	Refer to local podiatry service for further assessment.
	Screen every 6–12 months
High:	
Previous ulceration or	Provide foot care education.
Previous amputation or	Advise the person not to perform their own foot care.
On renal replacement therapy or	
Neuropathy & PAD together	Refer to local podiatry service for further assessment.
Neuropathy in combination with callus and/or deformity or	Screen every 1–3 months
PAD in combination with callus and/or deformity	
Active Diabetic foot problem	
Ulceration or	Refer within 1 working day to the multidisciplinary foot care service.
Infection or	
Chronic limb-threatening ischaemia or	
Gangrene or	For severe diabetic foot sepsis arrange for inpatient admission urgently within 24 hours.
Suspicion of an acute Charcot arthropathy, or an unexplained hot, swollen foot with a change in colour, with or without pain.	

Table 11.1 (*Contd.*)

Diabetic Foot Sepsis	
Red hot swollen foot—with or without ulceration	Refer immediately to acute services.
Foul smelling ulceration with purulent discharge	If an inpatient, refer to the MDT foot team urgently.
Suspected abscess-boggy collection upon palpation	
Rapidly worsening gangrene	If out of hours refer to local protocols
Spreading cellulitis	
Systemic signs of sepsis	

Neuropathy

Diabetic neuropathy is defined as nerve damage caused by high blood glucose levels. There are 3 types of neuropathy which in combination are referred to as polyneuropathy:

- Sensory—damage to the nerves that detect pressure, pain, heat and vibration
- Autonomic—affects autonomic body functions such as blood pressure, temperature control, digestion, bladder control and even sexual function
- Motor—nerves to the muscles can become damaged resulting in small muscle wasting within the foot leading to foot deformity.

Sensory neuropathy or loss of protective sensation (LOPS) affects 11–50% of people with diabetes[2] and should be assessed with one of the following techniques:

- Pressure perception: Semmes-Weinstein 10g monofilament
- Vibration perception: 128 Hz tuning fork
- When a monofilament or tuning fork are not available touch the toes test[6] can be performed with no equipment required.

Touch the Toes Test. (See Fig. 11.5):

- Ask the person to close their eyes and keep them closed until the end of the test
- Inform the person that you are going to touch their toes and ask them to say 'right' or 'left' as soon as they feel the touch depending on which foot has been touched
- Perform the touch using your index finger
- The diagram below shows the six toes which should be touched and in which order
- When the person responds, document 'Y' or 'N' if the touch has been felt correctly
- If two or more touches are not felt, then sensation is impaired.

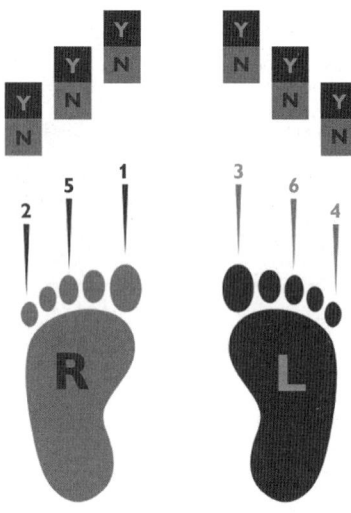

The subject's right foot,
as seen on your left

The subject's left foot,
as seen on your right

Fig. 11.5 Example of a Touch the Toes Test.

Image created by Alex Charlton of the Medical Illustration Department, Manchester University Foundation Trust NHS.

Case Study 1: Mr J

A 53 year old male with type 1 diabetes went on holiday to Dubai with his family in August, he was unaware that he had dense peripheral sensory neuropathy and walked with his family on the hot sand. It was one of his children who later noticed the damage to his feet, Mr J was completely unaware of the damage.

Upon arriving home after the holiday Mr J was admitted under the burns team at his local hospital and underwent a right 2nd toe amputation. A few weeks later whilst at home he felt very unwell and took himself to A & E.

Upon referral to the diabetic foot MDT it was clear that the right foot was not salvageable due to extensive bone infection and a week later the Mr J sadly had a below knee amputation. This case demonstrates the devastating affect of unknown sensory neuropathy and why education is so important in terms of prevention.

Patient A: Mr J

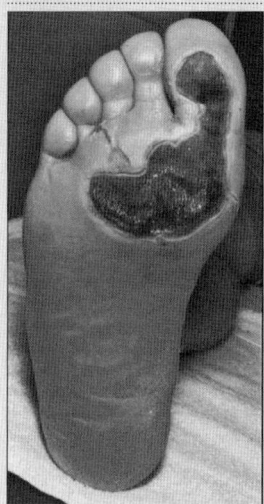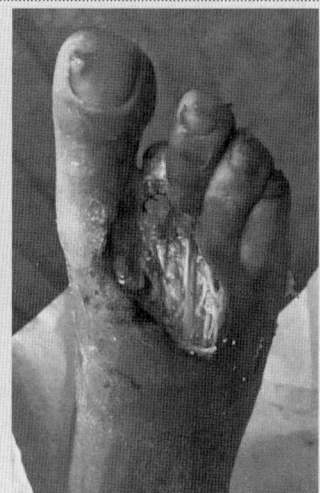

Photo used with written consent
Image available to view in colour on 🔗 https://academic.oup.com/
oxford-medicine-online

Upon returning from holiday	Post 2nd toe amputation—non viable wound bed with exposed bone visible

Peripheral Arterial Disease

Peripheral arterial disease (PAD) is a common condition that leads to the reduction of blood flow to the legs and feet. Diabetes is linked to extensive below the knee arterial disease which can be difficult to treat. Diabetic foot ulcers require adequate circulation to heal, if a person with diabetes also has PAD and develops a foot ulcer then the risk of amputation increases

PAD can be categorized into chronic and acute limb ischaemia[7]:

Chronic limb ischaemia:

- *Intermittent Claudication*—poor circulation which presents as pain in the lower limb when walking or during exercise that is relieved by rest.
- *Critical limb ischaemia*—severe impairment with imminent risk of limb loss.
- *Chronic limb-threatening ischaemia*—describes clinical patterns of varying degrees of ischaemia with or without tissue loss.

Acute Limb Ischaemia:
Sudden decrease in perfusion which develops over less than 2 weeks. The 6 P's is the acronym are used to recognise acute limb ischaemia:
- Pain
- Pallor
- Pulselessness
- Paralysis
- Paraesthesia
- Perishingly cold

Symptoms of PAD
- Hair loss to legs and feet
- Numbness or weakness in the legs
- Brittle, slow-growing toenails
- Ulcers (open sores) to feet and legs, which do not heal
- Changing leg skin colour e.g. pallor or blueness—this may be harder to see on brown and black skin
- 'Shiny' skin
- In men, erectile dysfunction
- The muscles in the legs shrinking (wasting)
- Intermittent claudication—sharp pain within buttocks, thighs or calf muscles when walking—alleviated by rest
- Rest pain—unable to sleep with the limb elevated

Assess for PAD if the person:
- Has symptoms suggestive of peripheral arterial disease, or
- Has diabetes, non-healing wounds on the legs or feet, or unexplained leg pain, or
- Is being considered for interventions to the leg or foot, or
- Needs to use compression hosiery.

NICE[4] recommends that any person who presents with a non-healing wound should be assessed for the presence of arterial disease. Ideally this assessment should be performed first and foremost using a handheld doppler by an experienced clinician.

An ankle brachial pressure index (APBI) is a measure of the ratio between the brachial pressure and the ankle pressure. A toe pressure is the measure of perfusion to the distal aspect of the foot and is the preferred measurement of distal flow if available.

If a doppler is not available, then the clinician can perform a basic hands on vascular assessment until further assessment is arranged.

Hands on vascular assessment:
- Palpation of foot pulses
- Temperature gradient
- Colour
- Capillary refill

Palpation of foot pulses

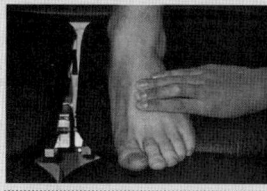 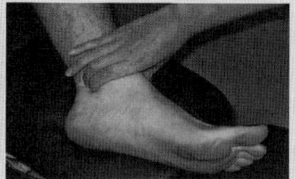

Photo used with written consent
Image available to view in colour on ♫ https://academic.oup.com/
oxford-medicine-online

DPA: Dorsalis Pedis	PTA: Posterior Tibia
Between the 1st and 2nd meta-tarsal bones	Behind medial malleolus

Introducing the WiFi classification system:

The Society of Vascular Surgery have developed a classification system to calculate the risk of amputation for people who present with tissue loss and ischaemia.

This system considers the three main compounding factors that threaten limb viability, wound, ischaemia and foot infection and is known as WiFi.[8]

This system can be downloaded as an app on most smartphones which is particularly useful when liaising with vascular teams (see figure 11.6).

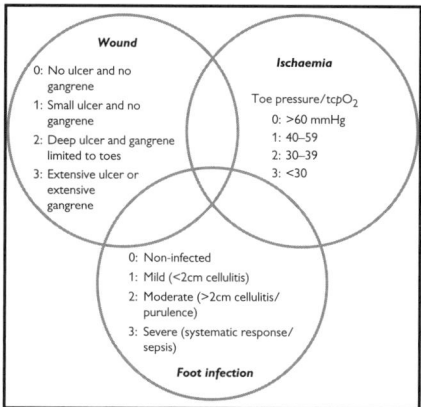

Fig. 11.6 Classification system to calculate the risk of amputation in people presenting with tissue loss and ischaemia.

Diabetic foot sepsis

Diabetic foot sepsis is a limb threatening and potentially life-threatening condition which should be treated as an emergency. Diabetic foot ulcers are highly susceptible to infection which can spread rapidly causing overwhelming tissue destruction. In such cases **'time is tissue'** whereby the longer the delay in receiving appropriate treatment the more tissue is lost.

It is essential that diabetic foot sepsis is recognised, and swift action is taken.

Signs of diabetic foot sepsis:
- Red hot swollen foot—with or without ulceration
- Foul smelling ulceration with purulent discharge
- Suspected abscess-boggy collection upon palpation
- Rapidly worsening gangrene
- Spreading cellulitis
- Systemic signs of sepsis

If it is suspected that a person has any of the above signs or symptoms refer urgently to the local A & E department for admission to hospital.

If the person is already an inpatient, then refer immediately (within 24 hours) to the inpatient multidisciplinary foot care service.

It is imperative that HCPs caring for those with diabetes are familiar with local foot care pathways

Examples of severe diabetic foot sepsis can be seen in the four cases below:

Case Study 2:

Patient B—This was a 37 year old male who was unable to attend his local podiatry follow up and presented at A & E due to feeling systemically unwell. Unfortunately due to the delay in seeking medical attention this led to a partial foot amputation

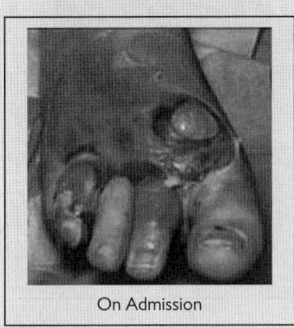

On Admission

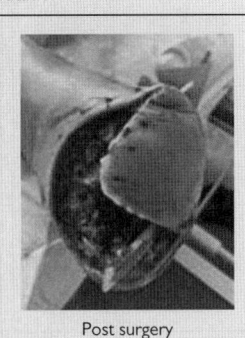

Post surgery

Photo used with written consent

Image available to view in colour on ᒭ https://academic.oup.com/oxford-medicine-online

Case Study 3:

Patient C was under the care of his high risk foot team who promptly referred him for hospital admission when his foot deteriorated. He was revascularised and had a 5th ray amputation.

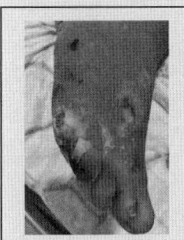

On admission to hospital

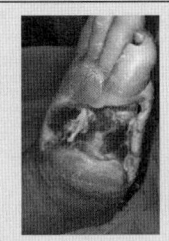

Upon discharge to home

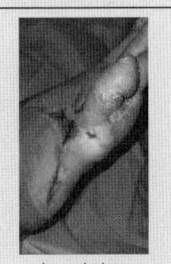

4 months later

Photo used with written consent

Image available to view in colour on ᒭ https://academic.oup.com/oxford-medicine-online

Case Study 4:

Patient D was admitted to hospital with a combination of diabetic foot sepsis and critical limb ischaemia. This patient underwent revascularisation followed by a partial foot amputation.

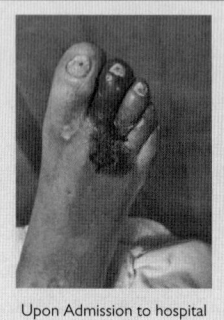
Upon Admission to hospital

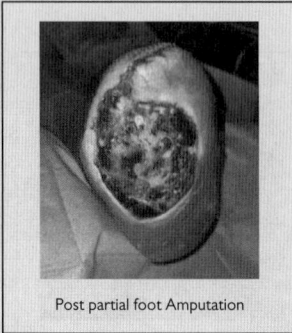
Post partial foot Amputation

Photo used with written consent

Image available to view in colour on 🕭 https://academic.oup.com/oxf ord-medicine-online

Case Study 5:

Patient E was initially seen by his GP with a superficial foot ulcer, he was prescribed oral antibiotics but there was no referral to his local high risk foot team but to his local treatment room which he waited 2 weeks for an appointment. During this time his foot condition had significantly deteriorated and his daughter was so concerned that she called an ambulance.

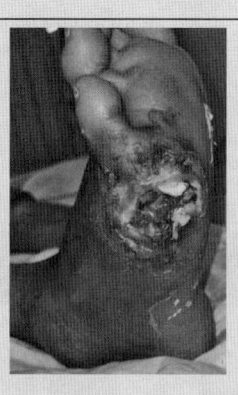 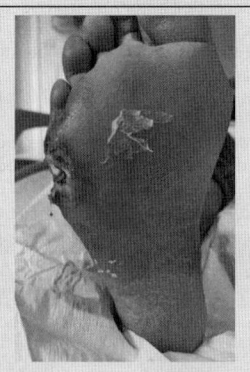

| Upon Admission to Hospital | Note the tracking erythema indicative of a deep collection |

Photo used with written consent

Image available to view in colour on 🔗 https://academic.oup.com/oxford-medicine-online

This gentleman was admitted to hospital with diabetic foot sepsis. Upon admission he was promptly referred to the inpatient diabetic foot team who arranged urgent scans and for the vascular team to review as he required urgent incision and drainage to remove the infected tissue.

The early signs of soft tissue infection can be difficult to spot in people with darker skin, clinicians need to be mindful of this and pay special attention to other signs such as swelling, heat and pain.

For further information on recognising diabetic foot infection, the author would suggest accessing the wounds UK consensus document 'Demystifying infection in the diabetic foot' which can be accessed online at: 🔗 https://wounds-uk.com/consensus-documents/demystifying-infection-in-the-diabetic-foot/

Foot ulcer prevention

Upon admission to hospital all people with diabetes should have a foot assessment and this should be documented clearly within a person's notes.

Educational tools

iDeal Diabetes is a multidisciplinary team which aims to improve education and awareness for people with diabetes and to reduce variation in care[10]. The 'ACT NOW' tool was developed as a simple tool for clinicians working with people with diabetes. By the widespread use of this tool, the iDeal diabetes team aim to reduce unnecessary amputation. The ACT NOW cards are credit card sized ideal to fit into a wallet or purse for easy reference for the person with diabetes. Cards have been translated into different languages and there are cards for different skin tones.

When to ACT NOW:
- **A** Recent or history of an accident or trauma?
- **C** Is there any new swelling, redness, change of shape of the foot?
- **T** If there is a change in temperature present? Infection or possible Charcot?
- **N** Is there new pain present? Is it localised or generalised throughout the foot?
- **O** What colour is any exudate (oozing)? Is there any odour?
- **W** document the size, shape and position of the wound in the foot affected.

The ACT NOW assessment tool is illustrated below:

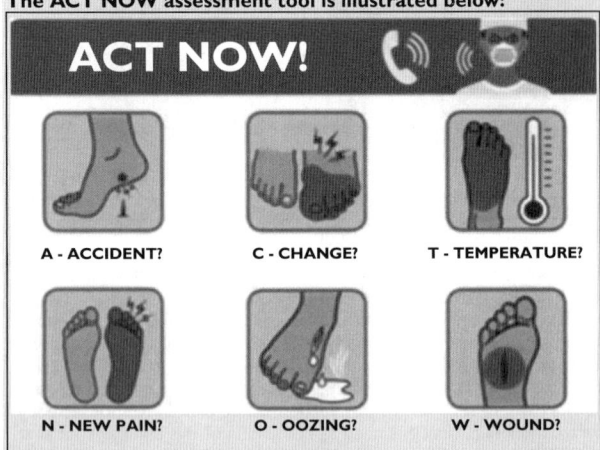

Available at: 🖰 **https://idealdiabetes.com/**

Foot care education

It is well documented that education plays a key role in reducing the incidence of diabetic foot ulcers.

Education should be provided at every clinician encounter to reinforce knowledge and to empower people with diabetes to engage and recognise potential foot problems early.

Diabetes UK has produced a 'top ten tips' leaflet[11] for people living with diabetes.

The Top Tips are:
- Get help to quit smoking
- Manage your blood sugars, cholesterol and blood pressure

- Check your feet every day
- Eat a healthy, balanced diet and stay active
- Watch out cutting your nails
- Make sure your footwear fits
- Use moisturising cream every day
- Don't use blades or corn plasters
- Get expert advice as necessary
- Keep useful numbers handy

Podiatry provision: foot care services

National guidance from NICE[4] recommends that all NHS Trusts have robust and clear pathways between foot care services.

The foot protection team is a podiatry led community service which aims to prevent diabetic foot problems and may treat and manage mild diabetic foot complications. These teams should have access to:
- Biomechanics & orthoses
- Wound care
- Diabetology

Should a person develop a moderate to severe diabetic foot ulcer then they should be referred onto their local multi-disciplinary foot care team.

The multi-disciplinary foot team

Effective management of diabetic foot ulcers requires an MDT effort focusing on neuropathy, PAD and infection.

NICE[4] stipulates that all people with active diabetic foot ulcers should have access to a MDT foot team. This team should consist of the following:
- Diabetology
- Podiatry
- Diabetes specialist nursing
- Vascular surgery
- Microbiology
- Orthopaedic surgery
- Biomechanics and orthoses
- Interventional radiology
- Casting
- Wound care

In addition, the MDT should have access to rehabilitation services, plastic surgery, psychological services and nutritional services.

People who present with active foot ulceration that is not deemed as diabetic foot sepsis should be referred to the MDT foot team within 1 working day.

Treatment of diabetic foot ulcers

It is beyond the scope of this chapter to fully explain all the treatment options for diabetic foot ulceration however the key principles of treatment are listed below:[12]
- Treatment of infection—either oral or intravenous antibiotics depending on the severity. This relies on the collection of a tissue sample from the wound or a deep wound swab.

- Assessment of blood supply, if compromised the vascular team will require further assessments & treatment planning.
- Debridement—the removal of dead tissue, this can be done by podiatrists using scalpel or surgically if extensive removal is required.
- Off-loading—to reduce the pressure. Gold standard recommendations is the application of an irremovable below knee cast followed by a below knee walker, sandal and insole.
- Application of appropriate dressings.
- Optimisation of blood glucose levels.

Summary

A key point to remember is that if a HCP is ever unsure of what action to take when a person presents with a diabetic foot problem, they should contact their local podiatry team without delay who will be able to advise.

Remember that '**time is tissue**' and any unnecessary delay could be the difference between limb salvage or amputation.

References

1. Kerr M, Rayman G, Jeffcoate WJ. Cost of diabetic foot disease to the national health service in England. *Diabetic Medicine*. 2014;**31**(12):1498–1504.
2. Edmonds M, Manu C, Vas P. The current burden of diabetic foot disease. *Journal of Clinical Orthopaedics and Trauma*. 2021 Feb 8;**17**:88–93. doi:10.1016/j.jcot.2021.01.017. PMID: 33680841; PMCID: PMC7919962.
3. Rogers L, Andros G, Caporusso J, et al.; Toe and Flow: Essential components and structure of the amputation prevention team. *Journal of Vascular Surgery*. 2010;**52**(3).
4. NICE (2016). Diabetic foot problems: prevention and management. NICE guideline (NG19), https://www.nice.org.uk/guidance/ng19
5. International Working Group on the Diabetic Foot (2019). Practical Guidelines on the prevention and management of diabetic foot disease. https://PracticalGuidelinesonthepreventionandmanagementofdiabeticfootdisease(IWGDF2019update)(iwgdfguidelines.org)
6. Ipswitch toes the toes test: Rayman, Rayman, G, Prashanth R. Vas, Neil Baker, Charles G. Taylor, Catherine Gooday, Amanda I. Alder, Mollie Donohoe; The Ipswich Touch Test: A simple and novel method to identify inpatients with diabetes at risk of foot ulceration. *Diabetes Care* 1 July 2011;**34**(7):1517–1518. https://doi.org/10.2337/dc11-0156
7. NICE CG147 (2012, Updated 2020). Peripheral arterial disease: Diagnosis & Assesment https://cks.nice.org.uk/topics/peripheral-arterial-disease/diagnosis/assessment/
8. Mills J, et al.; The Society for Vascular Surgery Lower Extremity Threatened Limb Classification System: Risk stratification based on Wound, Ischemia, and foot Infection (WIfI). *Journal of Vascular Surgery*. 2014;**59**(1). (2022) available at Accessed online: https://www.jvascsurg.org/article/S0741-5214(13)01515-2/fulltext
9. National diabetes foot care report— https://fingertips.phe.org.uk/static-reports/diabetes-footcare/national-diabetic-footcare-report.html
10. IDEAL Insights for Diabetes Excellence, Access and Learning (2020). *ACT NOW Assessment Tool*. Available at: https://idealdiabetes.com/act-now-education-resources/
11. Diabetes UK—How to look after your feet Available at: https://www.diabetes.org.uk/guide-to-diabetes/complications/feet/taking-care-of-your-feet#Know
12. Fletcher J, Edmonds M., Madden J, et al.; (2024). *Demystifying infection in the diabetic foot*. Wounds UK.

Diabetes-related eye disease, including retinopathy

There are two main ways in which diabetes can seriously affect the eyes:
- Diabetic retinopathy (DR)
- Diabetic macular oedema.

Diabetic retinopathy

Prevalence of diabetic retinopathy

DR is the most common form of eye disease among individuals with diabetes.[1]

DR was one of the leading causes of visual impairment and blindness in the UK among people of working age.[2] However, for the first time in five decades, diabetic eye disease has not been the main cause of sight-impaired registration (data from 2009 to 2010) because of regular diabetes screening programmes, improved glycaemic management, and new improved ophthalmic treatments such as intravitreal anti-vascular endothelial growth factor (VEGF) injections.[3]

A global meta-analysis (2021) of people with diabetes found that 22.27% had some form of DR, 17% had vision-threatening DR (VTDR), and 4.07% had clinically significant macular oedema (CSME).[4]

Risk factors for diabetic retinopathy

Modifiable	Non-modifiable
Glucose levels	Duration of diabetes
Blood pressure	Age
Lipid levels	Genetic predisposition
Smoking	Ethnicity

DR is a chronic and progressive disease which affects the retinal microvasculature due to hyperglycaemia and other associated risk factors.[2] The main measures to prevent visual loss include optimization of glycaemic levels (see ➲ Chapter 7), lipids and hypertensive management (see ➲ Chapter 10), and early identification of the retinopathy[5]

Grading of diabetic eye disease as per NHS Diabetic eye screening in England and Wales is shown in Table 11.2. Screening programmes and grading systems can be slightly different in Scotland and other different countries.[5]

Symptoms of diabetic retinopathy
- Gradual onset of blurred vision.
- Sudden loss of vision.
- Floaters.
- Patch of vision missing/blurred.

Table 11.2 Grading of diabetic eye disease (England and Wales)

R0	No retinopathy	Continue community screening
R1	Mild retinopathy	Continue community screening
R2	Moderate to severe Non-proliferative retinopathy	Routine referral to ophthalmology
R3	Proliferative retinopathy: R3A—active proliferative disease R3S—stable proliferative disease	Urgent referral to ophthalmology if active proliferation and routine referral if proliferation is stable
M0	No maculopathy	
M1	Maculopathy present	Routine referral to ophthalmology; however, if the combination is active proliferative retinopathy with maculopathy, then urgent referral to ophthalmology

Main types of diabetic retinopathy

- *Non-proliferative diabetic retinopathy (NPDR)*—this occurs in early stages of diabetic eye disease and can be asymptomatic. NPDR can be further classified as mild, moderate, and severe. It affects existing retina vessels, causing microaneurysms, retinal haemorrhages, exudates, and other retinal vascular changes, depending on severity.[6] No eye treatment is required, but regular monitoring with good glycaemic and CV risk factor management is essential.[2]
- *Proliferative diabetic retinopathy (PDR)* (see Figs 11.7 and 11.8)—this describes advanced changes due to diabetes; however, people can still be asymptomatic. Neovascularization (growth of abnormal blood vessels) and scar tissue form at the retina, causing haemorrhage, retinal detachment, and other visual deteriorations.[2]
- *Panretinal photocoagulation (PRP) laser*—this is used to treat retinal neovascularization and retinal ischaemia.[1] Intravitreal anti-VEGF injection or a combination of both laser and intravitreal injection (IVI) is given to some persons, depending on severity and response to treatment.[6]

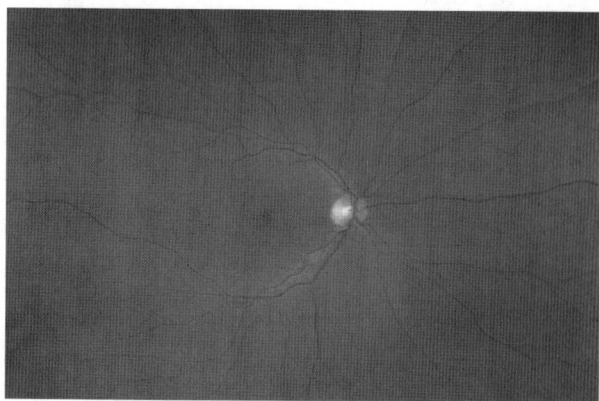

Fig. 11.7 Photo of the fundus of a normal retina vasculature in the right eye of a person with type 2 diabetes (photo used with written consent).

Image available to view in colour on ℬ https://academic.oup.com/oxford-medicine-online

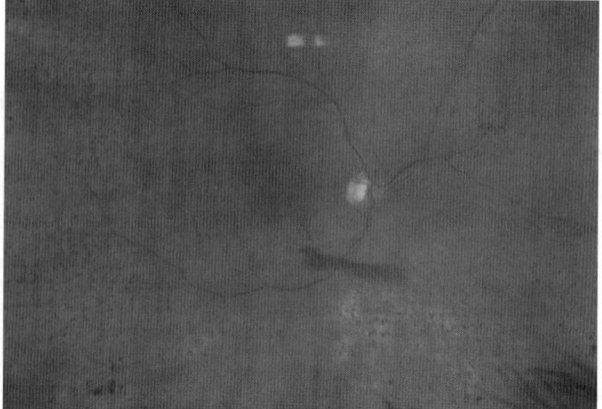

Fig. 11.8 Photo of the fundus in treated proliferative diabetic retinopathy in the right eye of a person with type 2 diabetes with suboptimal glycaemic levels (photo used with written consent).

Image available to view in colour on ℬ https://academic.oup.com/oxford-medicine-online

Surgical procedures such as vitrectomy, removal of scar tissue, and retinal re-attachment may be needed, depending on presentation and complications.[1]

Treatment options for diabetic retinopathy
(See Table 11.3)

Table 11.3 Treatment options for diabetic retinopathy	
Panretinal photocoagulation laser	The aim is to treat areas of the peripheral retina with laser. This treatment stops the retina from producing growth factors that stimulate new blood vessels to grow
Anti-VEGF injection	This is given by injection into the eye and is a course of treatment with people likely to need several injections at repeated intervals
	Drugs that are used to block the action of a chemical called VEGF. These injections try and prevent new vessels from growing and shrink the ones that have formed[1]
Surgery	If a severe bleed occurs due to bleeding new vessels, sometimes an operation is required to remove the blood and vitreous jelly in the eye.[3] Scarring at the retina can cause tractional retinal detachment, which needs retinal reattachment surgery

Diabetic maculopathy

The macula is the central part of the retina which is responsible for de-
tailed central vision and colour vision.[2] Damaged macular microvasculature
makes blood vessels leak fats and fluid into the macula that are normally
carried along in the bloodstream.[1] Fats that are leaked are called exudates,
and leaking fluid causes oedema at the macula.[6] Occasionally, blood vessels
can become narrow, which deprives the macula of oxygen and nutrients,
causing ischaemic maculopathy.[1]

Symptoms of diabetic maculopathy
- Early stages often asymptomatic.
- Central visual blurring.
- Central scotoma (blind spot/patch in central vision).
- Colour vision impairment.

Treatment for diabetic maculopathy
Treatment depends on the location and extent of macular thickening
(see Table 11.4).[2] Optical coherence tomography (OCT) helps to assess
macular thickness for management and treatment (Figs 11.9 and 11.10).

Table 11.4 Treatment for diabetic maculopathy as per location and extent of macular thickening

Presentation/findings		Treatment
Centre-involving macula oedema	400 microns and above	Anti-VEGF intravitreal injection, steroid intravitreal injection
	<400 microns	Optimize glycaemia and look to CVD risk reduction
Non-centre-involving macula oedema	Potential to get worse or affecting vision	Focal macula laser

VEGF, vascular endothelial growth factor; CVD, cardiovascular disease.

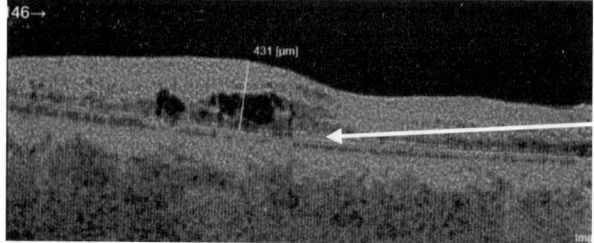

Fig. 11.9 Optical coherence tomography scan showing the normal macula of a person with optimized type 2 diabetes (photo used with written consent).

Image available to view in colour on ℛ https://academic.oup.com/oxford-medicine-online

Fig. 11.10 Optical coherence tomography scan showing diabetic maculopathy with diabetic oedema (measuring >400 microns) of a person with non-optimized type 2 diabetes (photo used with written consent).

Image available to view in colour on ℛ https://academic.oup.com/oxford-medicine-online

Different treatment options for diabetic maculopathy
(See Table 11.5.)

Table 11.5 Treatment options for diabetic maculopathy

Anti-VEGF injection	VEGF is produced in excess in eyes suffering from diabetic macular oedema and plays a role in the development of leakage from retinal blood vessels. The most used anti-VEGF drugs are Vabysmo® (faricimab) and Eylea® (aflibercept).[1] On rare occasions, biosimilar ranibizumab or bevacizumab may also be considered
Ozurdex® (short-acting steroid implant injected in the same way as anti-VEGF injections)	If the fluid does not respond well enough to anti-VEGF injections or if anti-VEGF is deemed unsuitable, steroid injections will be considered in the management plan.[1] As the implant slowly dissolves in the vitreous gel, it releases the steroid for up to 6 months
Iluvien® (long-lasting steroid injection/implant)	It is longer-acting than Ozurdex®. It releases the drug over a period of up to 3 years[6]
Localized macula laser	Laser can be used to treat vessels leaking away from the centre of the macula. Fluorescein angiography can be used to identify the leaking points

Other ocular pathology in undiagnosed or non-optimized diabetes

- Uveitis: new-onset uveitis (ocular inflammation) presents with a red, painful eye and blurred vision. It can be unilateral or bilateral. Most of these cases resolve with topical corticosteroid therapy, in addition to diabetes optimization.[2]
- Dry eyes.
- Poor healing of corneal ulcers/abrasions.
- Early onset of cataract.
- Extraocular muscle palsies: a person may present with binocular diplopia, and vascular conditions are one of the causes of muscle palsies such as diabetes, hypertension, and hypercholesterolaemia.[2]
- Neovascular glaucoma: proliferative diabetic retinopathy can also cause iris and anterior chamber angle neovascularization, which blocks fluid from draining out of the eye, causing glaucoma.[2]
- Diabetic papillopathy: a rare ocular manifestation, which can be seen in both people with type 1 diabetes (T1D) and those with T2D of all ages.[7] Rapid improvement in glycaemic levels is thought to be associated with diabetic papillopathy. Once all other life-threatening causes of optic disc oedema have been ruled out, observation is a reasonable initial approach, as most people improve with gradual glycaemic and other vascular risk factor optimization.[7]

Prevention of diabetic eye disease

- Optimization of glycaemic levels based on individualized targets (see ➲ Chapters 7 and 10).
- Optimization of blood pressure and lipids.
- Reduction in progression results in a better prognosis than treatment.

- Regular diabetic eye screening as per local and national protocols.
- Smoking cessation where appropriate.
- For implications in pregnancy,[8] see ➔ Chapters 14 and 15.

References

1. Teo ZL, Tham YC, Yu M, *et al*. Global prevalence of diabetic retinopathy and projection of burden through 2045: systematic review and meta-analysis. *Ophthalmology*. 2021;**128**(11):1580–91.
2. Salmon JF. *Kanski's Clinical Ophthalmology: A Systematic Approach*, 9th edition. Elsevier, 2019. Available at: 🔗 https://shop.elsevier.com/books/kanskis-clinical-ophthalmology/salmon/978-0-7020-7711-1
3. Mathur R, Bhaskaran K, Edwards E, *et al*. Population trends in the 10-year incidence and prevalence of diabetic retinopathy in the UK: a cohort study in the clinical practice research datalink 2004–2014. *BMJ Open*. 2017;**7**(2):e014444.
4. Teo ZL, Tham YC, Yu M, *et al*. Global prevalence of diabetic retinopathy and projection of burden through 2045: systematic review and meta-analysis. *Ophthalmology*. 2021;**128**(11):1580–91. Available at: 🔗 https://pubmed.ncbi.nlm.nih.gov/33940045/
5. Varma DR (2020). *NHS Diabetic eye screening (DES) programme* (gpraj). Available at: 🔗 https://gpraj.com/ophthalmology/2020/1/4/diabetic-eye-screening
6. Ockrim Z, Yorston D. Managing diabetic retinopathy. *BMJ*. 2010;**341**:c5400. Available at: 🔗 www.bmj.com/content/341/bmj.c5400
7. Pineda-Garrido E, *et al*. Diabetic papillopathy: two cases. *Neurology Perspectives*. 2021;**1**(4):244–6. Available at: 🔗 www.elsevier.es/en-revista-neurology-perspectives-17-articulo-diabetic-papillopathy-two-cases-S2667049621000594
8. National Institute for Health and Care Excellence (2015, updated 2020). *Diabetes in pregnancy: management from preconception to the postnatal period*. NICE guideline [NG3]. Available at: 🔗 www.nice.org.uk/guidance/ng3

Diabetic autonomic neuropathy

Diabetic autonomic neuropathy (DAN) has been defined as a disorder of the autonomic nervous system in the setting of diabetes or metabolic derangements of pre-diabetes after exclusion of other causes.[1]

Major clinical manifestations of diabetic autonomic neuropathy

- Resting tachycardia.
- Orthostatic hypotension.
- Gastroparesis.
- Constipation.
- Diarrhoea.
- Faecal incontinence.
- Erectile dysfunction (ED) (see ➲ Erectile dysfunction, p. 182).
- Neurogenic bladder.
- Sudomotor dysfunction with either ↑ or ↓ sweating.

Screening for symptoms of autonomic neuropathy includes asking about symptoms of:
- Orthostatic intolerance (dizziness, light-headedness, or weakness with standing)
- Syncope
- Exercise intolerance
- Constipation
- Diarrhoea
- Urinary retention
- Urinary incontinence
- Changes in sweat function.

Further testing can be considered if symptoms are present and will depend on the end organ involved, but might include CV autonomic testing, sweat testing, urodynamic studies, gastric emptying, or endoscopy/colonoscopy.[2]

Cardiac autonomic neuropathy

Treatment of symptomatic orthostatic hypotension includes:
- Optimization of glycaemic levels and CVD risk reduction
- Stopping drugs that may worsen symptoms
- Volume correction
- Strength training
- Pharmacological therapy, which may include fludrocortisone.

Gastrointestinal autonomic neuropathy

This includes gastroparesis (delayed gastric emptying).

The ADA[3] recommends evaluating for gastroparesis in people with diabetic neuropathy, retinopathy, and/or nephropathy by assessing for symptoms of:
- Unexpected glycaemic variability
- Early satiety
- Bloating
- Nausea
- Vomiting.

Management

- Referral to specialist MDTs, including a specialist dietitian.
- Ensuring adequate nutrition, as many people with gastroparesis (around 60%) consume fewer calories than is recommended.
- Trial of low-fat, low-fibre, small-particle, or liquid diets.
- Nutritional supplements.
- Enteral feeding may be required for relief of symptoms and/or to meet ongoing nutritional needs in some people.
- Optimization of glycaemic levels.
- Optimal insulin management for people with T1D, including consideration for pump or hybrid closed loop therapy (see ➜ Chapter 6).
- Pharmacological therapies that may be used include:
  - Dopamine receptor antagonists
  - Motilin receptor agonists
  - Other antiemetics.

References

1. Tesfaye S, Boulton AJ, Dyck PJ, et al.; Toronto Diabetic Neuropathy Expert Group. Diabetic neuropathies: update on definitions, diagnostic criteria, estimation of severity, and treatments. Diabetes Care. 2010;**33**:2285–93.
2. Sharma JK, Rohatgi A, Sharma D. Diabetic autonomic neuropathy: a clinical update. Journal of the Royal College of Physicians of Edinburgh. 2020;**50**(3):269–73.
3. American Diabetes Association Professional Practice Committee. 9. Pharmacologic approaches to glycemic treatment: standards of care in diabetes—2024. Diabetes Care. 2024;**47**(Suppl 1):S158–78.

Erectile dysfunction

(See ➐ Chapter 14 for ♀ sexual dysfunction.)

ED is when a person is either unable to get an erection or unable to sustain an erection for long enough to have sex.

ED is over three times more common in men with diabetes than in those without diabetes, affecting >50% of men with diabetes.[1]

The pathophysiology of ED in diabetes may be multifactorial, including neurological and vascular impairment.

It important to note that T2D is associated with androgen deficiency, so men living with T2D should be screened for any testosterone deficiency and managed accordingly, should their testosterone levels be lowered.[2]

Research by Diabetes UK has highlighted that despite the raised prevalence of ED in diabetes, only 15–20% of men advised that they were asked about this during their annual diabetes review.[1]

Risk factors

- Diabetes.
- Metabolic syndrome.
- Older age.
- Sedentary lifestyle.
- Living with obesity.
- Dyslipidaemia.
- Vascular disease.
- Smoking.
- Certain medications are also associated with ED such as:
    - Diuretics
    - Anticholinergics
    - Antidepressants
    - Hormone treatment
    - Cytotoxic agents/chemotherapy
    - Some antihypertensives.

Diagnosis

(See Fig. 11.11)

Management

The primary objective in the management of ED is to enable the man/couple to enjoy a satisfactory sexual experience.

Consider the efficacy, safety, and contraindications of different treatments, and the person's and partner's preferences

Treat any modifiable/potential risk factors, for example:

- Smoking cessation where appropriate
- Alcohol reduction where appropriate
- Optimise HbA1c (see ➐ Chapter 7)
- Optimise lipids (see ➐ Chapter 10)
- Optimise blood pressure (see ➐ Chapter 10)
- Look to reduce CV risk (see ➐ Chapter 10)

Diagnosing Erectile dysfunction

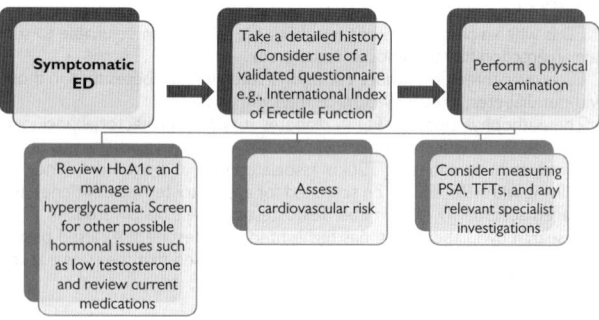

Hackett G, Kirby M, Wylie K et al (2018) British Society for Sexual Medicine guidelines on the management of erectile dysfunction inmen–2017. *JSex Med* 15: 430–57
https://www.baus.org.uk/_userfiles/pages/files/Patients/Leaflets/iief.pdf

Fig. 11.11 Diagnosing erectile dysfunction.

- Look to weight management interventions as appropriate (see ➲ Chapter 4)
- Optimise physical activity
- Review the use of any recreational drugs
- Review medications which may contribute to, or exacerbate, ED
- Consider referral for psychosexual/relationship therapy if appropriate
- Manage any abnormal testosterone levels, thyroid function tests, and prostate-specific antigen results.

First-line interventions
- Lifestyle and risk factor modification.
- For men not at high cardiac risk from sexual activity, a phosphodiesterase 5 (PDE5) inhibitor may be prescribed:
  - PDE5 inhibitors include sildenafil (Viagra®), tadalafil (Cialis®), vardenafil (Levitra®), and avanafil (Spedra®).
  - See the British National Formulary[3] and individual SMPCs for prescribing advice, including timing of taking the medication and any contraindications.
- Arrange for 6- to 8-week follow-up to assess response to treatment.
- Consider increasing to the maximum dose of the PDE5 inhibitor, depending on symptom response and adverse effects.
- Advise to try each PDE5 inhibitor 4–8 times at the maximum tolerated dose before switching to an alternative drug.
- Suggest a trial of at least two different PDE5 inhibitors taken sequentially before classing the person as a 'non-responder'.[4]

If PDE5 inhibitors or other treatment are ineffective, not tolerated, or contraindicated, offer referral to a urology specialist.

Second-line interventions (under the care of a specialist)
- Vacuum erection devices
- Intracavernous injection therapy, or
- Intraurethral alprostadil, or
- Alprostadil cream
- Vascular surgery/angioplasty
- Penile prosthesis.

When to consider referral

- To urology—for young men who have always had difficulty in obtaining or maintaining an erection; for men with a history of trauma (e.g. to the genital area, pelvis, or spine); if an abnormality of the penis or testicles is found on examination; and failure to respond as above to PDE5 inhibitors.
- To endocrinology—for men who have hypogonadism.
- To cardiology—for men who have severe/unstable CVD that would make sexual activity unsafe or be a contraindication to the use of PDE5 inhibitors.
- For mental health/psychological/relationship support—for men with an underlying psychogenic cause of ED and those with severe mental distress.[4]

References

1. Hackett G, Kirby M, Wylie K, *et al*. British Society for Sexual Medicine Guidelines on the management of erectile dysfunction in men—2017. *Journal of Sexual Medicine*. 2018;15(4):430–57. Available at: ℘ https://bssm.org.uk/wp-content/uploads/2023/02/BSSM-ED-guidelines-2018-1.pdf
2. Diabetes UK (2019). *Us, diabetes and a lot of facts and stats*. Available at: ℘ www.diabetes.org.uk/resources-s3/2019-11/facts-stats-update-oct-2019.pdf
3. British National Formulary (BNF) (2024). Available at: ℘ https://bnf.nice.org.uk
4. National Institute for Health and Care Excellence (2024). *Erectile dysfunction: scenario: management of erectile dysfunction*. Available at: ℘ https://cks.nice.org.uk/topics/erectile-dysfunction/management/management

Further reading

British Association of Urological Surgeons (2024). *Erectile dysfunction (impotence)*. Available at: ℘ www.baus.org.uk/patients/conditions/3/erectile_dysfunction_impotence
British Association of Urological Surgeons. *International Index of Erectile Function. Patient questionnaire*. Available at: ℘ www.baus.org.uk/_userfiles/pages/files/Patients/Leaflets/iief.pdf

Acute complications of diabetes

Hypoglycaemia

Hypoglycaemia is a lower-than-normal blood glucose concentration. It results from an imbalance between glucose supply, glucose utilization, and existing insulin concentration. It can be defined as 'mild' if the episode is self-treated and 'severe' if assistance is required.[1]

Hypoglycaemia is the commonest side effect of insulin or sulfonylurea therapy used to treat diabetes.

Definition

The National Institute for Health and Care Excellence (NICE) defines hypoglycaemia as a glucose value of <3.5mmol/L.[2] The American Diabetes Association describes three levels of hypoglycaemia based on recommendations by the International Hypoglycaemia Study Group (see Table 12.1).[3,4]

For people living with diabetes, hypoglycaemia may be better defined by the clinical picture and by the degree of distress and disruption an episode may cause.[5]

Table 12.1 Levels of hypoglycaemia as defined by International Hypoglycaemia Study Group

Name	Plasma glucose level	Implications
Hypoglycaemia alert	<3.9 mmol/L	• Lower limit of 'glucose in range' • Usually asymptomatic • Treat to prevent hypoglycaemia • Consider medication regimen change if recurrent
Clinically important	<3.0 mmol/L	• Associated with impaired cognitive function • Repeated episodes cause reduced hypoglycaemia awareness • Predicts severe hypoglycaemia • Associated with cardiac arrhythmias • Predicts mortality
Severe	Not specified	• Cognitive decline results in the need for treatment by another person • May be further divided to specify episodes requiring parenteral therapy and/or episodes associated with loss of consciousness or seizure

Prevalence
- For a variety of reasons, hypoglycaemia is often not reported.
- A recent meta-analysis showed that the prevalence of hypoglycaemia ranged from 0.074% to 73.0%, comprising a total of 2,462,810 individuals with diabetes.[6]

Potential impacts of hypoglycaemia
(See Fig. 12.1)
- Psychological effects (fear of hypoglycaemia).
- Reduction in quality of life.
- Physical morbidity (blackouts, seizures, coma, cognitive dysfunction).
- Cardiovascular damage (cardiac arrhythmias, ischaemic heart disease).
- Adherence challenges with treatment (defensive snacking and weight gain, suboptimal glucose management).
- Accidents and injury (fractures, road accidents).
- Economic costs (days off work, hospital admissions, ambulance callouts).[5]

Factors associated with increased risk of hypoglycaemia
Medical issues
- Stringent glycaemic management.
- Previous history of severe hypoglycaemia.
- Long duration of type 1 diabetes (T1D).
- Duration of insulin therapy in type 2 diabetes (T2D).
- Impaired awareness of hypoglycaemia.
- Severe hepatic dysfunction.
- Impaired renal function (including renal replacement therapy).
- Sepsis.

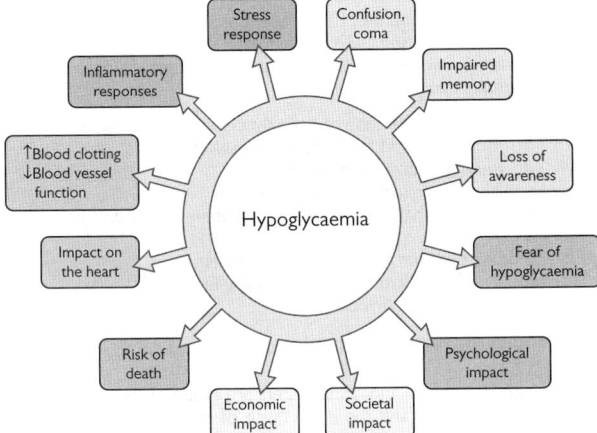

Fig. 12.1 The consequences of hypoglycaemia.[5]

- Terminal illness.
- Cognitive dysfunction/dementia.

Lifestyle issues
- ↑/unplanned exercise (relative to usual).
- Irregular lifestyle.
- Alcohol.
- ↑ age.
- Early pregnancy.
- Breastfeeding.
- No or inadequate blood glucose monitoring if taking a medication associated with hypoglycaemia e.g. sulfonylurea and/or insulin.

Carbohydrate intake/absorption
- Food malabsorption (e.g. gastroenteritis, coeliac disease, pancreatic exocrine insufficiency).
- Bariatric surgery involving bowel resection.

Prevention of hypoglycaemia

- Access to appropriate glucose monitoring if in a high-risk group (includes all persons taking a sulfonylurea and/or insulin).
- For people with T1D and some with T2D, offer continuous glucose monitoring (CGM) as per local and national guidance (see ⤵ Chapter 7).
- Empower/educate the person with diabetes where appropriate, to be able to self-titrate medication doses based on glucose levels.
- Appropriate management of glucose levels if missed meal/↑ activity.
- Appropriate intake of alcohol.
- Optimal injection technique and injection site rotation.
- Appropriate timing of medications.
- Easy access to hypoglycaemia treatment, even when away from home and when driving.
- Care homes, nursing homes, and inpatient areas to have access to a 'hypo' box for timely and appropriate treatment of low glucose levels.
- Timely diabetes reviews with healthcare team, particularly following any hypoglycaemic episode.

Useful questions for exploration of hypoglycaemia in consultations include:
- What do you understand by the term 'hypoglycaemia'?
- What do you think causes hypoglycaemia?
- How would you recognize hypoglycaemia?
- Have you ever felt shaky or sweaty, maybe when you haven't eaten for a while?
- Do you drive, cycle, or regularly operate machinery?
- Have you ever had a 'hypo' and how did you feel?
- How would you treat a 'hypo'?

Signs and symptoms of hypoglycaemia

(See Fig. 12.2)
Ensure that the person and family/carers are aware of the early warning signs of hypoglycaemia and the importance of immediate blood glucose measurement and emergency treatment of an acute episode.

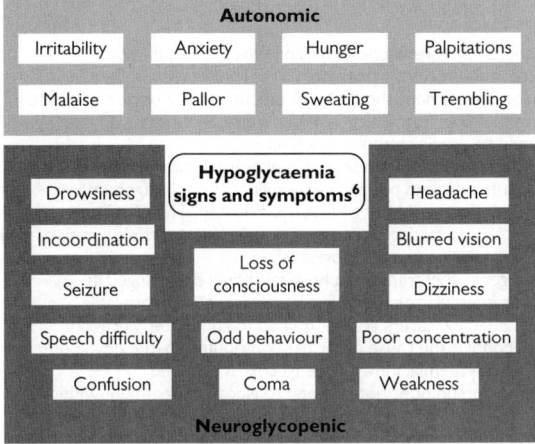

Fig. 12.2 Signs and symptoms of hypoglycaemia.

- In older persons, there is blunting of the physiological adrenergic responses (tremor, sweating, palpitations), which means that blood glucose levels fall further before the onset of symptomatic hypoglycaemia.
- In addition, neuroglycopenic manifestations (confusion, sleepiness, aggression) may be mistaken for cognitive impairment.
- Elderly/frail people will be more at risk from the consequences of hypoglycaemia such as the potential for falls and injury.

Treatment of hypoglycaemia

In adults who are conscious, orientated, and able to swallow:
- Give 15–20g of quick-acting carbohydrate:
  - 200mL (a small carton) of pure fruit juice
  - 60mL of Lift juice shot®
  - Five glucose tablets (e.g. Glucotabs®)
  - 5–7 dextrose tablets
  - Four large jelly babies
  - Two tubes of glucose gel (such as GlucoGel® or Dextrogel®).
- Recheck glucose level after 10–15 minutes; if the blood glucose level is <4mmol/L, repeat one of these treatments.
- Once the glucose level has risen to >4mmol/L, a starchy carbohydrate snack is recommended or a meal containing carbohydrate (if the hypo occurred prior to a meal). If no starchy carbohydrate is eaten following

the fast-acting carbohydrate 'hypo treatment', the glucose level will start to fall again.

In adults who are unconscious and unable to swallow:
- Place in the recovery position.
- Glucose treatment should NOT be put into the person's mouth.
- Intramuscular (e.g. GlucaGen®) or subcutaneous (e.g. Ogluo®) glucagon should be administered immediately.
  - Glucagon is contraindicated in phaeochromocytoma.
  - Cautious use in people with insulinoma or glucagonoma.
  - Not effective if liver glycogen is depleted. Thus, ineffective after prolonged fasting or if adrenal insufficiency, chronic hypoglycaemia, or alcohol-induced hypoglycaemia.
- Emergency 999 transfer to hospital should be arranged if:
  - Intramuscular or subcutaneous glucagon is not available.
  - The family/carers are not trained to administer glucagon.
  - Alcohol is the cause of, or has contributed to, the development of hypoglycaemia: intravenous glucose is required.
  - The person does not respond to glucagon treatment within 10 minutes—will require treatment with intravenous glucose.
- If the person responds to glucagon treatment within 10 minutes and is sufficiently alert and able to swallow safely, advise them to eat some oral carbohydrate.
- Vomiting is common in the recovery phase and hypoglycaemia may recur—close monitoring is required.

Impaired hypoglycaemia awareness

Impaired hypoglycaemia awareness is defined as reduced ability to recognize or perceive the onset of low blood glucose levels.

Validated questionnaires, such as the Clarke, Gold, and Pedersen tools, are useful methods to assess impaired hypoglycaemia awareness and can be clinically important in identifying people with T2D who may benefit from CGM.[7]

For driving regulations, see ➲ Chapter 17.

References

1. British National Formulary (2022). Hypoglycaemia. Available at: ℗ https://Bnf.Nice.Org.Uk/Treatment-Summary/Hypoglycaemia.Html
2. National Institute for Health and Care Excellence, Clinical Knowledge Summaries (CKS) (2021). *Scenario: Insulin therapy – type 2 diabetes.* Available at: ℗ https://cks.nice.org.uk/topics/insulin-therapy-in-type-2-diabetes/management/insulin-therapy-type-2-diabetes/#hypoglycaemia
3. American Diabetes Association. Standards of medical care in diabetes – 2022. Abridged for primary care providers. *Clinical Diabetes.* 2022;**40**:10–38.
4. International Hypoglycaemia Study Group. *What is hypoglycaemia?* Available at: ℗ www.ihsgonline.com/what-is-hypoglycaemia-2
5. Amiel SA. The consequences of hypoglycaemia. *Diabetologia.* 2021;**64**:963–70.
6. Alwafi H, Alsharif AA, Wei L, *et al.* Incidence and prevalence of hypoglycaemia in type 1 and type 2 diabetes individuals: a systematic review and meta-analysis. *Diabetes Research and Clinical Practice.* 2020;**170**:108522.
7. Alkhatatbeh MJ, Abdalqader NA, Alqudah MAY. Impaired awareness of hypoglycaemia in insulin-treated type 2 diabetes mellitus. *Current Diabetes Reviews.* 2019;**15**:407–13.

Hospital management of hypoglycaemia

Most hypoglycaemic episodes occur in people admitted to hospital for another reason—it is quite unlikely to be the primary cause of admission. Hypoglycaemia was the reason for admission in only 5% of admissions for people with T1D and 1.5% of admissions for people with T2D.[1]

Based on data from National Diabetes Inpatient Audit (NaDIA),[2] almost 1 in 5 patients with diabetes have a hypoglycaemic episode during their hospital stay. The main reason for this could be related to the tendency to maintain tighter glycaemic levels in hospitalized patients. Fig. 12.3 shows the distribution of hypoglycaemic episodes experienced by people with diabetes in hospital.[2]

- Mortality rates are found to be higher in hospitalized patients with hypoglycaemia. Studies have shown that people remain in hospital for 4.1 days longer if they experience hypoglycaemia, with almost double the risk of in-hospital mortality.[3]
- Hypoglycaemia episodes can lead to ↑ length of stay and health costs.

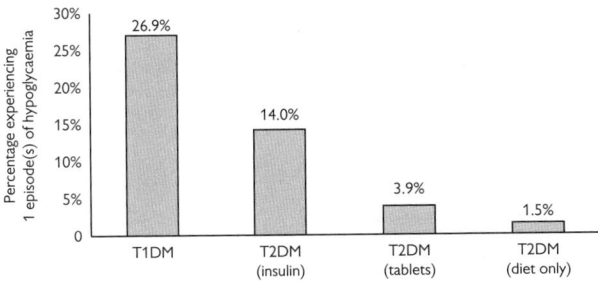

Fig. 12.3 Percentage of people experiencing ≥1 episode of hypoglycaemia in hospital?

Definition

All non-pregnant adults with diabetes in hospital should be treated if the blood glucose level is <4.0mmol/L.[4]

- In view of ↑ mortality rate in people experiencing hypoglycaemia in hospitals, glucose targets have been relaxed to ensure patient safety. Hence, a blood glucose level of between 4.0 and 6.0mmol/L could indicate 'looming hypoglycaemia', particularly if these episodes are occurring more frequently.
- Review of current diabetes treatment is required to identify the need for any dose adjustments in these patients.[4]
- There should be a personalized approach as a blood glucose level of between 4.0 and 6.0mmol/L could be an individualized target range for some patients.
- Early involvement with the inpatient diabetes team is important in formulating a personalized diabetes management plan in this group of patients.

References

1. Pratiwi C, Mokoagow MI, Kshanti IAM, Soewondo P. The risk factors of inpatient hypoglycemia: a systematic review. *Heliyon*. 2020;**6**:e03913.
2. NaDIA. National Diabetes Inpatient Audit 2019 [Internet]. 2020. Available from: ℞ https://digi tal.nhs.uk/data-and-information/publications/statistical/national-diabetes-inpatientaudit/2019
3. Lake A, Arthur A, Byrne C, Davenport K, Yamamoto JM, Murphy HR. The effect of hypogly-caemia during hospital admission on health-related outcomes for people with diabetes: a system-atic review and meta-analysis. *Diabetes Medicine*. 2019;**36**:1349–59.
4. Joint British Diabetes Societies for Inpatient Care (2023). *The hospital management of hypoglycaemia in adults with diabetes mellitus*. Available at: ℞ https://abcd.care/sites/default/files/site_uploads/ JBDS_Guidelines_Archive/JBDS_01_Hypo_Guideline_FINAL_23042021_Archive.pdf

Factors that can precipitate hypoglycaemia in hospitals
(See Fig. 12.4)

Insulin Prescription Errors	Medical Issues	Carbohydrate intake issues
• Inappropriate use of 'stat' or 'PRN' rapid/short-acting insulin (i.e. repeated doses of rapid- acting insulin without leaving sufficient time between to allow for onset of action and duration of effect) • Confusing the insulin name with the dose (e.g. Humalog Mix25 becoming Humalog 25 units) and insulins with similar sounding names (e.g. Novorapid & Novomix 30) • Confusing the concentration with the dose (be very careful if dose is written as 100units, it could be the insulin concentration instead which is usually 100units per ml) • Only insulin syringes should be used to withdraw insulin from a vial, syringes used for intravenous administration should never be used for insulin. • Inappropriately withdrawing insulin using a standard insulin syringe (100units/ml) from prefilled insulin pens containing higher insulin concentrations (e.g. 200units/ml or 300 units/ml) • Misreading poorly written prescriptions – when 'U' is used for units (i.e. 4U becoming 40 units); always write 'UNITS' in full • Confusion regarding the indications for prescription of glucose and insulin infusion to control blood glucose and a glucose and insulin infusion for hyperkalaemia treatment (i.e. 50units in 50ml sodium chloride 0.9% instead of 10units of insulin with 25g glucose) • Incorrect drug history and failure to correctly reconcile on admission	Acute discontinuation of long-term corticosteroid therapy • Recovery from acute illness/stress • Mobilisation after illness • Major amputation of a limb • Incorrect type of insulin or oral hypoglycaemia therapy prescribed and administered • Inappropriately timed insulin or oral hypoglycaemia therapy in relation to meal or enteral feed • Change of insulin injection site • IV insulin infusion with or without glucose infusion • Inadequate mixing of intermediate-acting or mixed insulins • Regular insulin doses or oral hypoglycaemia therapy being given in hospital when these are not routinely being taken at home • Failure to monitor blood glucose adequately whilst on IV insulin infusion	Missed or delayed meals • Less carbohydrate than normal • Change of the timing of the biggest meal of the day (i.e. main meal at midday rather than evening) • Lack of access to usual between meal or before bed snacks • Prolonged starvation time e.g. 'Nil by Mouth' • Vomiting • Reduced appetite • Reduced carbohydrate intake • Omitting glucose while on IV insulin infusion

Fig. 12.4 Potential causes of hypoglycaemia in hospital.[1]

Treatment

Some hospitals have a provision of 'hypo boxes', which contain a good supply of rapid-acting treatments. The introduction of 'hypo boxes' has shown an ↑ in appropriate management of hypoglycaemic episodes from 42% to 82%.[2] (See Fig. 12.5 for the image of a 'hypo box'.)

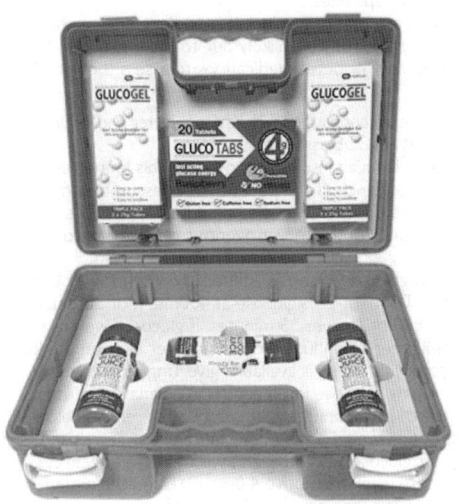

Fig. 12.5 Image of a 'hypo box'.

Hypoglycaemia treatment options depend upon the level of consciousness of the patient.

1. Adults who are conscious, orientated, and able to swallow:
- If the patient is on an insulin infusion, stop this immediately.
- Give 15–20g of rapid-acting carbohydrate. Rapid-acting treatment options available in a hospital setting include:
  - 5–7 dextrose tablets
  - One bottle (60mL) of Lift juice shot®
  - 150–200mL of pure fruit juice.
- Repeat capillary blood glucose measurements every 10–15 minutes, and repeat the rapid-acting treatment if the glucose level is still <4.0mmol/L.
- If the blood glucose level remains <4.0mmol/L after three cycles of rapid-acting treatment, call for medical assistance.
- Once the glucose level is above 4.0mmol/L, give a long-acting carbohydrate snack (15–20g). Long-acting treatment options available in a hospital setting include:

- Two biscuits
- One slice of bread/toast
- 200–300mL glass of milk
- Normal meal if due (must contain carbohydrate).
- If the patient was on intravenous insulin, adjust the insulin rate and ensure a glucose infusion is running concurrently to prevent further hypoglycaemic episodes.
- Do not omit any regular insulin injection dose due, as the hypoglycaemic episode is unlikely due to the insulin which is about to be given. Review diabetes medications to assess the need for dose reductions.

2. *Adults who are unconscious and/or having seizures and/or are very aggressive:*
- Complete an ABCDE assessment.
- If the patient is on an insulin infusion, stop this immediately.
- Check local guidance. If the patient has a rescue treatment prescription already available, administer the prescribed treatment, which will usually be a prescription of intravenous glucose and/or intramuscular glucagon.
- Intravenous glucose is used as a first option if intravenous access is available—100mL of 20% glucose at 400mL/h or 200mL of 10% glucose at 800mL/h over 15 minutes. If glucose levels remain below 4.0mmol/L after 15 minutes, repeat another infusion of glucose.
- If no intravenous access is available, give 1mg of glucagon intramuscularly. Glucose levels return to normal limits usually after a single dose of glucagon treatment, but if they remain below 4.0mmol/L, the best option would be to obtain intravenous access and administer an intravenous glucose infusion as this will be more effective.
- Once glucose levels are above 4.0mmol/L and the patient has recovered, give a long-acting carbohydrate snack.
- If the patient was on intravenous insulin, adjust the insulin rate and ensure a glucose infusion is running concurrently to prevent further hypoglycaemic episodes.
- Do not omit any regular insulin injection dose due, as the hypoglycaemic episode is unlikely due to the insulin which is about to be given. However, review diabetes medications to assess the need for dose reductions.

3. *Adults who are nil by mouth:*
- Complete an ABCDE assessment.
- If the patient is on an insulin infusion, stop this immediately.
- Intravenous glucose is used as a first option if intravenous access is available. Options are to give 100mL of 20% glucose at 400mL/h or 200mL of 10% glucose at 800mL/h over 15 minutes. If glucose levels remain below 4.0mmol/L after 15 minutes, repeat another infusion of glucose.
- Assess the need for starting a variable-rate intravenous insulin infusion once blood glucose levels are above 4.0mmol/L, especially if the patient is to remain nil by mouth.

4. Adults requiring enteral/parenteral feeding:
- Complete an ABCDE assessment.
- If the patient is on an intravenous insulin infusion, stop this immediately.
- Give 15–20g of rapid-acting carbohydrate via an enteral feeding tube:
  - One bottle of Lift juice shot®
  - 150–200mL of fruit juice
  - 50–70mL of Fortijuice® (NOT Fortisip)
- All treatments should be followed by a 40–50mL water flush of the feeding tube to prevent tube blockage.
- Restart the enteral/parenteral feed to rapidly deliver 15–20g of carbohydrate.
- Repeat capillary blood glucose measurement in 15 minutes, and if still <4.0mmol/L, repeat the rapid-acting treatment.
- If the capillary blood glucose level remains <4.0mmol/L after three cycles of rapid-acting treatment, administer intravenous glucose.
- Do not omit any regular insulin injection dose due, as the hypoglycaemic episode is unlikely due to the insulin which is about to be given. But review diabetes medications to assess the need for dose reductions.

Once hypoglycaemia is successfully treated:
- Complete the National Diabetes Inpatient Safety Audit (NDISA) if the patient required injectable rescue treatment for the management of hypoglycaemia.[3]
- Restock 'hypo boxes' as appropriate.
- Review local guidance, and ensure that the patient would benefit from a rescue treatment prescription of intravenous glucose and/or intramuscular glucagon, which can be used 'as needed'.
- Identify and treat risk factors for hypoglycaemia.
- Refer the patient to the inpatient diabetes team for advice and guidance.
- Do not treat isolated spikes of hyperglycaemia with additional doses of rapid-acting insulin.
- Ensure the patient has adequate glucose monitoring equipment for home, and provide hypoglycaemia management education with a supply of written resources such as leaflets.[4]

References

1. Joint British Diabetes Societies for Inpatient Care (2023). The hospital management of hypoglycaemia in adults with diabetes mellitus. Available at: ℘ https://abcd.care/sites/default/files/site_uploads/JBDS_Guidelines_Archive/JBDS_01_Hypo_Guideline_FINAL_23042021_Archive.pdf

2. Livingstone R, Boyle J. Improving the quality of assessment and management of hypoglycaemia in hospitalised patients with diabetes mellitus by introducing 'hypo boxes' to general medical wards with a specialist interest in diabetes. *BMJ Quality Improvement Reports*. 2015;**4**:u207686.w3067.

3. NHS England. *National Diabetes Inpatient Safety Audit*. Available at: ℘ https://digital.nhs.uk/data-and-information/clinical-audits-and-registries/national-diabetes-inpatient-safety-audit

4. Trend Diabetes (2023). *Diabetes: Why do I sometimes feel shaky, dizzy and sweaty? Hypoglycaemia explained*. Available at: ♒ https://trenddiabetes.online/portfolio/diabetes-why-do-i-sometimes-feel-shaky-dizzy-and-sweaty-hypoglygaemia-explained/

Further reading

EDEN. *A helping hand with hypos*. Available at: ♒ https://static1.squarespace.com/static/5a6439bab7411c94f2ebe216/t/633fe6b8cc9395486e97c896/1665132217196/Helping_Hand_with_Hypos_Infographic.pdf

Diabetic ketoacidosis

Diabetic ketoacidosis (DKA) is a serious life-threatening complication of diabetes caused by an absolute or relative absence of insulin. It occurs commonly in people with type 1 diabetes (T1D) but can also develop in people with type 2 diabetes (T2D) in the presence of extreme stress such as severe sepsis, trauma, and cardiovascular or other emergencies.[1] DKA is a medical emergency and must be treated intensely. Depending on the severity of DKA, a person may require the critical care unit or high dependency unit for intensive monitoring.

DKA can also be the first presentation for a person with new-onset T1D.

Coronavirus disease 2019 (COVID-19) infections led to an ↑ in DKA episodes in both people with T1D and those with T2D due to severe insulin resistance and dehydration.

Pathophysiology

Lack of insulin and the presence of counter-regulatory hormones, such as cortisol, glucagon, and catecholamines, can lead to ↑ gluconeogenesis and lipolysis. This causes hyperglycaemia, which then leads to osmotic diuresis, dehydration, and impaired renal function. Lipolysis causes the conversion of free fatty acids to ketone bodies, which then leads to ketoacidosis. Urinary excretion of ketones coerces sodium and potassium loss, which also causes severe dehydration[1] (see Fig. 12.6[2]).

Precipitating causes

- New diagnosis of T1D.
- Acute illness.
- Missed, omitted, or forgotten insulin doses.
- Medical, surgical, or emotional stress.
- Insulin pump malfunction.
- Psychological problems such as eating disorders or substance misuse.
- Sodium–glucose cotransporter 2 (SGLT2) inhibitor therapy (see ➔ Chapters 2 and 17).

Signs and symptoms

- Dry skin and tongue.
- Smell of ketones (fruity smell of acetone).
- Nausea and vomiting.
- Abdominal pain/tenderness.
- Hypotension.
- Osmotic symptoms such as polyuria and polydipsia.
- Kussmaul respirations (laboured breathing).
- Altered level of consciousness.

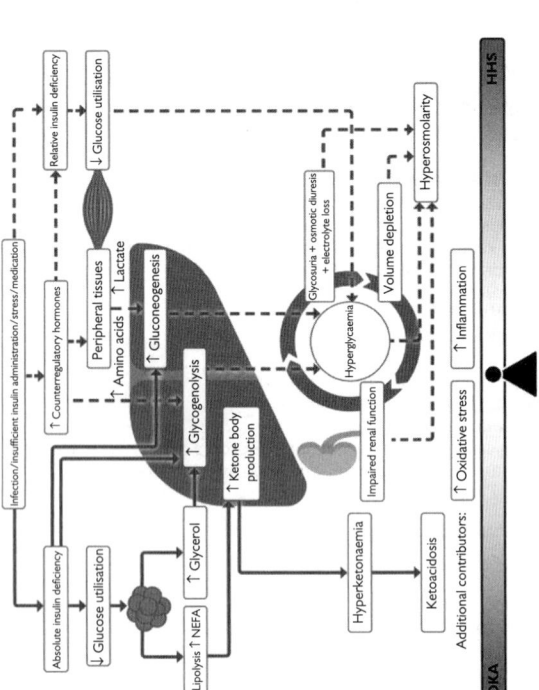

Fig. 12.6 Pathogenesis of DKA and HHS.
Umpierrez, G.E., Davis, G.M., ElSayed, N.A. et al. Hyperglycaemic crises in adults with diabetes: a consensus report. Diabetologia (2024). © https://doi.org/10.1007/s00125-024-06183-8

Diagnosis

The diagnostic criteria for DKA are:[2]

Diabetes/hyperglycaemia	Glucose ≥11.1mmol/L (200mg/dL) OR prior history of diabetes
Ketosis	Blood ketone concentration ≥3.0mmol/L OR urine ketone strip 2+ or greater
Metabolic acidosis	pH <7.3 and/or bicarbonate concentration <15.0mmol/L

Differential diagnosis

Euglycaemic diabetic ketoacidosis

This is a condition characterized by euglycaemia (normal blood glucose levels), severe metabolic acidosis, and ketonaemia. This mainly occurs in people undergoing prolonged starvation due to conditions such as anorexia, gastroparesis, fasting, use of ketogenic diet, and ↑ use of alcohol. Other precipitating factors are pregnancy, pancreatitis, surgery, sepsis, and use of illicit drugs such as cocaine.

Introduction of the new group of oral diabetes medication known as SGLT2 inhibitors has shown an ↑ in euglycaemic DKA (EDKA) episodes in people with T2D, although this remains a rare adverse event. SGLT2 inhibitors are also used in the management of chronic kidney disease (CKD) and heart failure (HF) in people without diabetes (see ➜ Chapter 10).

Conditions such as pregnancy, sepsis, surgery, trauma, major illness, persistent vomiting, reduced diet intake, and suboptimal diabetes management can trigger the presence of EDKA. EDKA can occur in people with T1D. SGLT2 inhibitors are not licensed for use in T1D[3] (see ➜ Chapters 2 and 10).

Ketosis-prone type 2 diabetes

DKA can also occur in people with ketosis-prone T2D. This is a rare type of diabetes that has been observed in people of Afro-Caribbean or Hispanic descent. Although the pathogenesis is not fully understood, it is believed to be caused by stress-induced, but reversible, pancreatic β-cell dysfunction. People will exhibit ketosis without acidosis and require insulin therapy, but often come off insulin therapy quickly, especially when the underlying precipitating condition is treated (see ➜ Chapter 1).

Alcoholic ketoacidosis

Normal or slightly elevated glucose levels in the presence of ketoacidosis is the main feature of this condition. The person will reveal a recent history of binge drinking, reduced food intake, and persistent vomiting.

Starvation ketosis

Lack of carbohydrate intake is the main reason for this and is a condition that occurs gradually over several days. Reduced intake of carbohydrates can lead to reduction in insulin secretion, lipolysis, and subsequent ketosis. But the presence of acidosis is quite minimal, as the condition occurs over a prolonged period.

Management of all these conditions is similar to DKA management, with a slight exception to EDKA, which will be discussed in the next section.

Management of diabetic ketoacidosis

The main aspects of DKA management include:
- Correction of fluid loss with intravenous fluids
- Correction of hyperglycaemia with insulin
- Correction of electrolyte disturbances
- Correction of acid–base balance
- Treatment of precipitating factors
- Strict monitoring of glucose, ketone, and electrolyte levels.

The 2023 Joint British Diabetes Societies (JBDS) guidelines[4] recommend the use of crystalloids rather than colloids, with 0.9% sodium chloride solution (normal saline) as the preferred choice (see Table 12.2). The fluid rate may need to be modified in people with renal failure, those with HF, the elderly, and adolescents. Once the blood glucose level falls below 14mmol/L, a 10% dextrose infusion should be added concurrently to prevent hypoglycaemia. A fixed-rate intravenous insulin infusion is recommended, which is calculated as 0.1 units/kg body weight (see Table 12.3). Short- or rapid-acting insulin is used, and the infusion is made up of 50 units of insulin in 49.5mL of 0.9% sodium chloride solution. Many hospitals use pre-prepared insulin infusion syringes. If already on long-acting basal insulin, this must be prescribed and continued at the usual dose. For those with newly diagnosed diabetes, this must be prescribed at a dose of 0.25 units/kg subcutaneously once daily. If using an insulin pump, this should be stopped, removed and stored safely whilst on the DKA management pathway.

Table 12.2 Example of a fluid replacement regime

Fluid	Volume
0.9% sodium chloride 1L	1000mL over first hour
0.9% sodium chloride 1L with potassium chloride	1000mL over next 2 hours
0.9% sodium chloride 1L with potassium chloride	1000mL over next 2 hours
0.9% sodium chloride 1L with potassium chloride	1000mL over next 2 hours
0.9% sodium chloride 1L with potassium chloride	1000mL over next 2 hours
0.9% sodium chloride 1L with potassium chloride	1000mL over next 2 hours

JBDS-IP (2023). The Management of Diabetic Ketoacidosis in Adults, Joint British Diabetes Societies for Inpatient Care. Revised March 2023.

Table 12.3 Example of calculating insulin dose for weight

Weight (kg)	Insulin dose per hour (units) at 0.1 units/kg/hour if glucose >14mmol/L
40–49	4
50–59	5
60–69	6
7–79	7
80–89	8
90–99	9
100–109	10
110–119	11
120–130	12
130–139	13
140–150	14
>150	15 (any dose higher than this should be on the advice of the diabetes specialist team)

JBDS-IP (2023). The Management of Diabetic Ketoacidosis in Adults, Joint British Diabetes Societies for Inpatient Care. Revised March 2023.

Metabolic targets

Recommendations are:[4]

- Fall in capillary blood glucose levels by 3.0mmol/L/hour
- Fall in blood ketone levels by 0.5mmol/L/hour
- ↑ in venous bicarbonate levels by 3.0mmol/L/hour
- Maintain potassium levels between 4.0 and 5.5mmol/L.

Blood glucose and ketone levels must be monitored hourly.

Fixed-rate intravenous insulin infusion rate must be ↑ if the above targets are not achieved.

Reduce insulin rate to 0.05 units/kg/hour to avoid hypoglycaemia if glucose levels are falling rapidly.

Management of euglycaemic diabetic ketoacidosis

The two main differences in managing EDKA vs DKA are:

- Addition of 10% dextrose, along with 0.9% sodium chloride, right from the beginning as glucose levels generally be <14mmol/L.
- Reduce insulin rate to 0.05 units/kg/hour to avoid hypoglycaemia if glucose levels are falling rapidly.

SGLT2 inhibitors must be discontinued, and a 'Yellow Card' should also be completed. In most cases, these drugs are not restarted due to ↑ risk of developing EDKA in the future.

All patients admitted with DKA or EDKA must be referred to the diabetes specialist team to improve patient safety, deliver education, reduce length of hospital stay, prevent recurrence, and facilitate appropriate follow-up.

Table 12.4 Example of potassium replacement guidance

Potassium level in first 24 hours (mmol/L)	Potassium replacement (mmol/L) of infusion solution
Over 5.5	Nil
3.5–5.5	40
Below 3.5	Senior review as additional potassium needs to be given

JBDS-IP (2023). The Management of Diabetic Ketoacidosis in Adults, Joint British Diabetes Societies for Inpatient Care. Revised March 2023.

Complications of diabetic ketoacidosis

Hypokalaemia and hyperkalaemia

During the initial stages of DKA, a normal or raised potassium level may be seen due to the extracellular shift of potassium in the presence of acidosis, and potassium levels will start to fall with insulin therapy, leading to hypokalaemia. Potassium of 40mmol/L must be added to 0.9% sodium chloride solution if potassium levels are below 5.5mmol/L (see Table 12.4). Local policies must be in place to ensure hyperkalaemia management is done safely.

Hypoglycaemia

With the introduction of fixed-rate intravenous insulin infusion, glucose levels will start to fall, and this could lead to severe hypoglycaemia if glucose levels are not monitored appropriately. Hence, it is important to commence 10% dextrose to run alongside 0.9% sodium chloride when glucose levels fall below 14mmol/L. In patients with EDKA, the rate of 10% dextrose infusion may need to be ↑ if glucose levels are falling despite a reduction of insulin rate to 0.05 units/kg/hour.

Cerebral oedema

Cerebral oedema causing symptoms is relatively uncommon in adults, but any changes in Glasgow Coma Scale score should be addressed immediately with urgent management and imaging. Urgent treatment with mannitol or hypertonic saline should be commenced rapidly.[5]

Resolution of diabetic ketoacidosis

- Capillary ketone level <0.6 mmol/L.
- Venous pH over 7.3.

Once this is achieved, check if the person is eating and drinking. If not managing oral intake, convert fixed rate intravenous insulin infusion to variable rate intravenous insulin infusion. If oral intake is established, convert the fixed-rate intravenous insulin infusion to a subcutaneous insulin regime. Subcutaneous insulin regime conversion must ideally be commenced by the diabetes specialist team, especially in patients with newly diagnosed diabetes. Hence, it is vital for hospital teams to provide daily diabetes team cover to allow anyone admitted with DKA to be reviewed within 24 hours of their admission.

Case study 1: diabetic ketoacidosis

Joe, 20 years old, was admitted to the emergency department (ED) feeling generally unwell, extremely tired, and thirsty over the last few days. Started vomiting the previous day and has been struggling to take food and fluids orally. Attended general practice surgery in the morning, no access to blood ketone monitoring, but urinalysis showed positive ++ for ketones. Advised to attend the ED. Denies intake of alcohol. Usually fit and healthy, plays football, attends gym 3–4 times per week. No history of any past medical illness. Grandfather has T2D, takes insulin therapy. Joe mentioned that he has lost a considerable amount of weight over the past 2–3 weeks without making any dietary changes or increasing his exercise. Clinical examination shows dry skin and tongue, and a slightly tender abdomen. Admission venous blood gas shows blood glucose level of 16.0mmol/L, pH of 7.27, bicarbonate level of 15.0, and blood ketone level of 4.8mmol/L.

Questions
1. What is wrong with Joe? What are your initial thoughts?
2. What are your immediate and long-term management plans? Think about safe discharge plans.

Answers
1. Joe is showing the classic symptoms of a new diagnosis of T1D and is also presenting with DKA (refer to the diagnostic criteria and symptoms of DKA).
2. Joe requires immediate fluid resuscitation and a fixed-rate intravenous insulin infusion. Blood samples must be sent for initial investigations such as full blood count, HbA1c, renal profile, C-reactive protein, random plasma glucose, and blood cultures. Urinalysis must also be performed. An ECG and a chest X-ray must be requested. Regular monitoring of metabolic targets must be followed to assess for resolution of DKA. Monitor for complications of DKA. Referral to the diabetes specialist teams must be done.

Once DKA has resolved, liaise with the diabetes specialist team about converting the fixed-rate intravenous insulin infusion to a subcutaneous insulin regime. The diabetes specialist team will facilitate training on the different aspects of T1D management such as insulin injection technique, hypoglycaemia management, care of insulin pens, glucose and ketone monitoring at home, access to technology, diet, and lifestyle management (see ➲ Chapters 3, 4, 5, and 6).

The diabetes specialist team will facilitate discharge from hospital once Joe can self-manage insulin therapy and glucose monitoring at home. Joe will be provided with adequate follow-up from the diabetes team post-discharge through regular telephone consultations. Follow-up appointments with various diabetes specialist teams, such as diabetes consultants, specialist nurses, and dietitians, will be arranged to facilitate long-term management of diabetes. Joe will receive further information, such as carbohydrate counting and sick day guidance, during regular appointments with them. See Table 12.5 for sick day guidance for people with T1D.[6]

Table 12.5 Sick day guidance for people with type 1 diabetes—if ketones less than 1.5 mmol/l. With Kind permission to use from TREND Diabetes

Glucose more than 11 mmol/L and/or you feel unwell, either with no ketones or blood ketones less than 1.5 mmol/L (negative or trace of urine ketones)

↓

Sip sugar-free fluids, at least 100 ml/hr. Eat as normal if possible. If not, see meal replacement suggestions (page 6). **You need food containing carbohydrate (carbs), insulin and fluids to avoid dehydration and prevent diabetic ketoacidosis**

↓

Test glucose and blood ketones
every 4 to 6 hours including during the night

↓

Aim to take your usual insulin dose. However, if your glucose is above 11 mmol/L, take additional insulin as below

↓

Glucose	Insulin dose
11–17 mmol/L	Add 2 extra units to each dose
17–22 mmol/L	Add 4 extra units to each dose
More than 22 mmol/L	Add 6 extra units to each dose
Call your GP or nurse if your glucose still remains higher than normal	

Sick day guidance for people with Type 1 diabetes—if blood ketones
1.5 mmol/l or higher. With Kind permission to use from TREND Diabetes

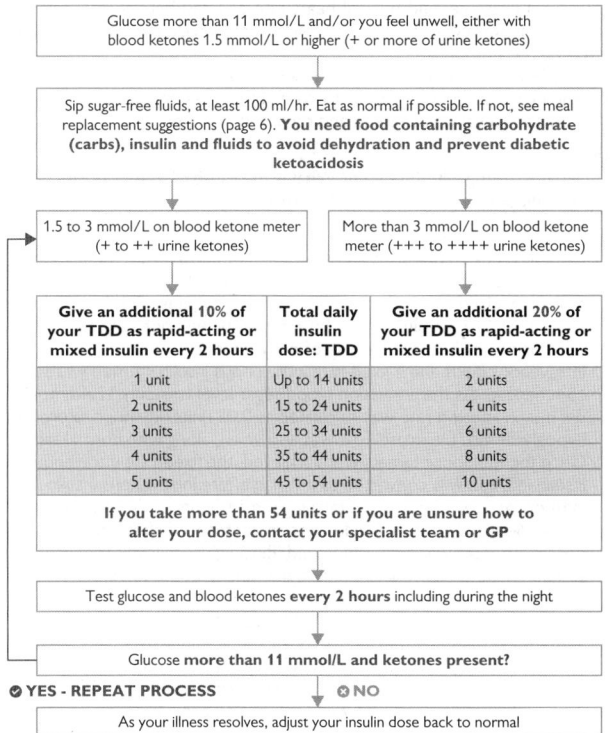

Glucose more than 11 mmol/L and/or you feel unwell, either with
blood ketones 1.5 mmol/L or higher (+ or more of urine ketones)

Sip sugar-free fluids, at least 100 ml/hr. Eat as normal if possible. If not, see meal
replacement suggestions (page 6). **You need food containing carbohydrate
(carbs), insulin and fluids to avoid dehydration and prevent diabetic
ketoacidosis**

1.5 to 3 mmol/L on blood ketone meter
(+ to ++ urine ketones)

More than 3 mmol/L on blood ketone
meter (+++ to ++++ urine ketones)

Give an additional 10% of your TDD as rapid-acting or mixed insulin every 2 hours	Total daily insulin dose: TDD	Give an additional 20% of your TDD as rapid-acting or mixed insulin every 2 hours
1 unit	Up to 14 units	2 units
2 units	15 to 24 units	4 units
3 units	25 to 34 units	6 units
4 units	35 to 44 units	8 units
5 units	45 to 54 units	10 units

**If you take more than 54 units or if you are unsure how to
alter your dose, contact your specialist team or GP**

Test glucose and blood ketones **every 2 hours** including during the night

Glucose **more than 11 mmol/L and ketones present?**

✓ YES - REPEAT PROCESS   ✗ NO

As your illness resolves, adjust your insulin dose back to normal

⚠ If you start vomiting, are unable to keep fluids down, or are unable to control
your glucose or ketone levels, you must seek urgent medical advice. DON'T
STOP TAKING YOUR INSULIN EVEN IF YOU ARE UNABLE TO EAT

Case study 2: euglycaemic diabetic ketoacidosis

Mrs John, a 64-year-old lady, attended the ED with diarrhoea and vomiting
over the last few days, lethargy, and minimal intake of diet and fluids. Medical
history of T2D, hypertension, and hypothyroidism. Takes metformin 1g
twice daily, gliclazide 160mg twice daily, and Dapagliflozin 10mg once daily.
Recent HbA1c 60mmol/mol. Fit and healthy normally.

Clinical examination on admission showed signs of dehydration, such as ↓ skin turgor and dry mucosa, and a tender abdomen. Vital signs showed low blood pressure, and normal heart rate and respiratory rate. Oxygen saturation recorded as 96% on room air. Admission capillary blood glucose level was 12.4mmol/L.

Initial blood results showed slightly elevated white blood cell count, acute kidney injury, and deranged electrolytes. Blood gas showed acidosis; pH <7.3. Ketone level was checked and recorded as 4.2mmol/L.

Questions

1. What is wrong with Mrs John? What is the cause of ketoacidosis?
2. How would you manage this effectively

Answers

1. Mrs John is exhibiting signs and symptoms of EDKA, with the presence of ketoacidosis and absence of hyperglycaemia. This is likely to be caused by diarrhoea and vomiting, and failing to pause SGLT2 inhibitor therapy. SGLT2 inhibitors must be withheld when not eating and drinking normally and/or at risk of dehydration.
2. Intravenous fluids and a fixed-rate intravenous insulin infusion were commenced. As the admission blood sugar level was only 12.4mmol/L, the insulin infusion rate was calculated as 0.05 units/kg/hour to prevent hypoglycaemia. Dextrose 10% was also given, along with normal saline. Once the metabolic targets were achieved, the fixed-rate intravenous insulin infusion was converted to a variable-rate intravenous insulin infusion, as Mrs John was not taking good amounts of diet and fluids orally. Metformin and gliclazide were recommenced after a few days once oral intake was fully established. Blood glucose levels remained within normal limits without adding any other glucose-lowering medications.

   Usual recommendation is to stop SGLT2 inhibitors in people admitted with EDKA, but as diarrhoea and vomiting may have been the precipitating factor for EDKA in Mrs John's case, the diabetes team requested the primary care team to consider restarting the SGLT2 inhibitor once Mrs John was well again and to provide access to blood ketone monitoring. Education on sick day guidance (see Table 12.6) was provided, including written information at discharge.[7]

Table 12.6 Sick day guidance for people taking SGLT2 inhibitors

- Stop taking SGLT2 inhibitors if unable to take good amounts of diet and fluids orally. This could be related to illness, infections, starvation, alcohol, surgery, diarrhoea, vomiting, and dehydration. Seek medical help if infection or illness.

- Suspect euglycaemic diabetic ketoacidosis if you have nausea, vomiting, abdominal pain, and difficulty with breathing, with glucose levels being normal or slightly elevated.

- Check blood ketone levels if you have ketone monitoring equipment at home, and if levels are above 0.6mmol/L, attend the local emergency department. If no ketone meter is available at home, present yourself for blood ketone testing at your local hospital.

- Drink plenty of water/sugar-free fluid to avoid severe dehydration.

- Do not restart SGLT2 inhibitors in people who developed euglycaemic diabetic ketoacidosis unless there was a clear precipitant which has been resolved.

References

1. Hirsch IB, Emmett M (2022). *Diabetic ketoacidosis and hyperosmolar hyperglycemic state in adults: Epidemiology and pathogenesis*. Available at: ℘ www.uptodate.com/contents/diabetic-ketoacidosis-and-hyperosmolar-hyperglycemic-state-in-adults-epidemiology-and-pathogenesis

2. Umpierrez GE, Davis GM, ElSayed NA, et al. Hyperglycaemic crises in adults with diabetes: a consensus report. *Diabetologia*. 2024;**67**:1455–79.

3. Medicines and Healthcare products Regulatory Agency (2021). *Dapagliflozin (Forxiga): no longer authorised for treatment of type 1 diabetes mellitus*. Available at: ℘ www.gov.uk/drug-safety-update/dapagliflozin-forxiga-no-longer-authorised-for-treatment-of-type-1-diabetes-mellitus

4. Joint British Diabetes Societies for Inpatient Care (2023). *The management of diabetic ketoacidosis in adults*. Available at: ℘ https://abcd.care/sites/default/files/site_uploads/JBDS_Guidelines_Current/JBDS_02_DKA_Guideline_with_QR_code_March_2023.pdf

5. Dhatariya KK, Glaser NS, Codner E, Umpierrez GE. Diabetic ketoacidosis. *Nature Reviews Disease Primers*. 2020;**6**:40.

6. Trend-UK (2020). *Type 1 diabetes: what to do when you are ill*. Available at: ℘ https://trenddiabetes.online/wp-content/uploads/2020/03/A5_T1Illness_TREND_FINAL.pdf

7. Dashora U, Patel D, Nagi D, et al. (2023). *SGLT-2 inhibitors in type 2 diabetes*. Available at: ℘ https://abcd.care/sites/default/files/resources/SGLT2-inhibitors-ABCD.pdf

Hyperosmolar hyperglycaemic state

Hyperosmolar hyperglycaemic state (HHS) is a clinical condition that mainly occurs in individuals with T2D. This was formerly known as hyperosmolar non-ketotic (HONK) coma. HHS is less common than DKA but is associated with a high mortality rate—as high as 20%, which is about 10 times higher than the mortality rate in DKA. It is a serious and potentially fatal complication of T2D and requires urgent medical attention. The main characteristics of HHS is hyperglycaemia, hyperosmolarity, and dehydration without significant ketoacidosis.[1]

Pathophysiology

The rise of counter-regulatory hormones, especially in conditions such as sepsis, cardiovascular insults including myocardial infarction and stroke, and certain medications including thiazide diuretics and glucocorticoids, can lead to a relative reduction in circulating insulin. Also, this may present in older persons being enterally fed with gradually rising hyperglycaemia and dehydration. Blood glucose levels start to rise, but the presence of small amounts of insulin inhibits lipolysis and ketosis. Hyperglycaemia leads to osmotic diuresis, which, in turn, causes electrolyte loss and severe dehydration (see Fig. 12.6). Dehydration is severe in patients with HHS due to loss of circulating water and often leads to hypovolaemia and shock if water loss is not compensated for by oral fluid intake. This can be difficult in frail elderly persons with other comorbidities; hence, it is crucial for a person to be admitted to hospital for intravenous fluid resuscitation and hyperglycaemia management.

Precipitating causes

- Infections (commonly, pneumonia and urinary tract infections).
- Acute events such as stroke, myocardial infarction, and acute pancreatitis.
- Patients with underlying renal disease and congestive HF.
- Drugs that cause hyperglycaemia such as alcohol, antipsychotics, β-blockers, diuretics, and corticosteroids.
- Omitting glucose-lowering medications.
- Parenteral and enteral nutrition.
- Dehydration.
- Acute kidney injury and CKD.

Signs and symptoms

- Polyuria and polydipsia.
- Fever.
- Altered mental status.
- Drowsiness and lethargy.
- Tachypnoea and tachycardia.
- Focal or generalized seizures.
- Visual changes or disturbances.
- Low Glasgow Coma Scale score.
- ↓ urine output.

Patients with HHS usually exhibit gradual onset of symptoms over a course of days to weeks.

Diagnosis

The diagnostic criteria for HHS are:[2]

H	**H**yperglycaemia	Plasma glucose ≥33.3mmol/l
H	**H**yperosmolarity	Calculated effective serum osmolality >300 mOsm/kg or total serum osmolality >320 mOsm/kg
S	Absence of **S**ignificant ketonaemia	β-hydroxybutyrate <3.0 mmol/l or urine ketones < 2+
	Absence of acidosis	pH ≥7.3 and bicarbonate concentration ≥15mmol/mol

Management

The main goals of HHS treatment are to:
- Normalize serum osmolality
- Replace fluid and electrolyte losses
- Normalize blood glucose levels
- Treat any underlying causes
- Monitor and assist cardiovascular, pulmonary, renal, and central nervous system (CNS) function.

Fluid losses must be corrected initially, and the rate of fluid replacement should be determined by assessing severity and any pre-existing comorbidities. Patients with HHS must be referred to the diabetes specialist team at the time of admission to hospital.

Treatment targets

- Sodium chloride 0.9% is the fluid of choice for rehydration.
- Insulin infusion must be started only if glucose levels are not falling despite intravenous fluid resuscitation. Fixed-rate intravenous insulin infusion is used at a rate of 0.05 units/kg/hour.
- Glucose levels must fall only at a rate of 5.0mmol/L per hour.
- Potassium replacement is similar to that used for DKA.
- Antibiotics must be given if there is clinical evidence of infection.
- Prophylactic low-molecular weight heparin must be given, unless contraindicated, to prevent venous thromboembolic disease.
- Foot risk assessment should be completed on admission to hospital to prevent foot ulceration, and every 24 hours thereafter. Appropriate mattress and heel protectors must be provided for those who are immobile.

Complications

Most frequent complications are electrolyte abnormalities such as hypokalaemia. Hence, it is important to monitor electrolytes frequently. Blood glucose levels must be checked closely, ideally every hour, to prevent sudden drop in blood glucose levels causing hypoglycaemia.[3] Cerebral oedema is also another fatal complication of HHS and can be identified by deterioration in the level of consciousness, lethargy, and headache. Cerebral oedema could be due to the sudden drop in plasma osmolality from osmotically driven movement of water into the CNS during treatment of HHS. Close monitoring of fluid balance and treatment targets are vital in preventing cerebral oedema.

Resolution of hyperosmolar hyperglycaemic state

- Calculated or measured serum osmolality falling to <300mOsm/kg.
- Correction of hypovolaemia.
- Improvement in cognitive status.
- Blood glucose <15mmol/L.

Resolution of HHS can take up to 72 hours, as this will be based on pre-existing health conditions, frailty, and management of precipitating factors. Once HHS is resolved and oral intake is well established, most people will need conversion of intravenous insulin to subcutaneous insulin. Patients must be reviewed by the diabetes specialist team for diabetes management and education, to prevent recurrence and to facilitate appropriate follow-up.[3]

The Clinical Features of DKA and HH

See Table 12.7

Table 12.7 Clinical features of DKA and HHS

Factors	DKA	HHS
Type of diabetes	Type 1	Type 2
Presentation	Rapid onset-hours	Gradual onset- days
pH	<7.3	>7.3
Serum Bicarbonate	<15	>15
Serum Ketone	>3.0 mol/L	<3.0 mmol/L
Serum Osmolality	<320mOsm/kg	>320mOsm/kg
Plasma Glucose typically	> 11 mmol/L	>30 mmol/L
Treatment	FRIII—0.1 units/kg/hr	Fluids initially and FRIII later if needed—0.05 units/kg/hr

Case study

Mr Singh, a 72-year-old gentleman, was brought to the ED with new onset of confusion, slurred speech, left-sided weakness, and swallowing difficulties. Medical history of T2D and hypertension. Glucose-lowering medications include metformin 1g twice daily, gliclazide 160mg twice daily, and sitagliptin 100mg once daily. Recent HbA1c was 100mmol/mol. His family confirmed that his blood glucose levels have been high at home, ranging between 12 and 30mmol/L.

Mr Singh appears lethargic, dehydrated, confused, and drowsy on admission. CT confirmed a diagnosis of ischaemic stroke. Admission blood glucose level was reported as 41.2mmol/L, with no presence of ketones. Blood gas showed no acidosis. Other blood results showed raised sodium (166mmol/L), urea (33.5mmol/L), creatinine, lactate, and C-reactive protein levels. Serum osmolality was calculated to be 396.7mOsm/kg ($[2 \times 166] + 41.2 + 33.5$), confirming the diagnosis of HHS.

An infusion of 0.9% sodium chloride was commenced immediately, and a fixed-rate intravenous insulin infusion was added after a few hours as there was no improvement in blood glucose levels. An ECG was obtained, and a chest X-ray confirmed pneumonia. Antibiotic therapy was added to treat chest sepsis. The fixed-rate intravenous insulin infusion was converted to variable rate, as blood glucose levels normalized after 12 hours and the patient was kept nil by mouth for bedside swallowing assessment. The patient was referred to the inpatient diabetes team for ongoing diabetes care and management.

Metabolic targets were achieved after 72 hours with intravenous fluids, insulin infusion, and antibiotics. Enteral feeding was commenced via a nasogastric tube, and the intravenous insulin infusion was converted to a subcutaneous insulin regime. Metformin and sitagliptin were reintroduced, and gliclazide was stopped in view of regular insulin therapy. Mr Singh needed a gastrostomy insertion after a few weeks due to impaired swallowing, and he was discharged to the stroke rehabilitation unit.

A referral was made to the local diabetes team and district nurses to provide support in the community with regard to long-term diabetes care and insulin management.

References

1. Avichal D (2024). *Hyperosmolar hyperglycemic state*. Available at: 🔗 https://emedicine.medscape.com/article/1914705-overview#a3

2. Umpierrez GE, Davis GM, ElSayed NA, *et al.* Hyperglycaemic crises in adults with diabetes: a consensus report. *Diabetologia*. 2024;**67**:1455–79.

3. Joint British Diabetes Societies for Inpatient Care (2022). *The management of hyperosmolar hyperglycaemic state (HHS) in adults*. Available at: 🔗 https://abcd.care/sites/default/files/site_uploads/JBDS_Guidelines_Current/JBDS_06_The_Management_of_Hyperosmolar_Hyperglycaemic_State_HHS_%20in_Adults_FINAL_0.pdf

Further Information about DKA and HHS

Prevention of DKA and HHS

A new consensus report published as the book went into print recommended[2]:

- Delivery of structured diabetes education programme
- Specific education on insulin administration and sick day guidance
- Adequate supply of diabetes resources at the time of hospital discharge such as insulin and glucose and ketone monitoring devices
- Providing contact information of diabetes health care professionals
- Address barriers to optimal self-management

The older person with diabetes

Introduction

There are an increasing number of older people living with diabetes, and their management may be different to that of the general population.[1]

Older does not necessarily mean frail, but there is often an overlap of frailty and end-of-life considerations for this group of people, including considering a person's ability to self-care and their social circumstances.

Many people living with advancing frailty have supported living, including residing in care homes and nursing homes or being assisted by community nurses/carers. Tasks such as insulin administration and glucose monitoring may or may not be supported.

It is essential that all social and health care practitioners have an understanding of diabetes, particularly in the key areas of:
- Hypoglycaemia
- Hyperglycaemia (including sick day guidance)
- Foot care
- Individualized glucose level targets (see Box 13.1; see ➲ Chapter 7).

This chapter highlights some of the additional considerations for this cohort of people who are living with diabetes and gives practical definitions, aims of treatment, and important factors to consider in care delivery.

Age-related changes can include:
- Cerebrovascular disease:
  - Transient ischaemic attack, stroke
  - Cognitive decline
  - Dementia (vascular and Alzheimer's).
- Coronary artery disease:
  - Angina
  - Myocardial infarction
  - Heart failure
- Peripheral arterial disease
- Peripheral neuropathy
- Chronic kidney disease
- Musculoskeletal disorders
- Mobility difficulties
- Falls
- Dizziness
- Sensory impairment
- Retinopathy
- Erectile dysfunction
- Incontinence
- Depression and anxiety
- Social isolation and loneliness
- Multimorbidity and polypharmacy
- Poor dentition
- Difficulty with mastication
- Sarcopenia
- Malnutrition

- Weight loss—likely due to poor oral intake
- Potential for vitamin D deficiency.

Reference

1. International Diabetes Federation (2021). *Diabetes Atlas*, 10th edition. Available at: ℜ https:// diabetesatlas.org/idfawp/resource-files/2021/07/IDF_Atlas_10th_Edition_2021.pdf

Frailty

The terms 'older' and 'frail' are often intertwined with each other, but they are not necessarily correlative[1] and it can be challenging to distinguish between the two.

When considering frailty, aside from age, Strain et al. (2021) suggested that it is a 'condition characterised by loss of biological reserves across multiple organ systems, and vulnerability to physiological decompensation after a stressor event'.[1]

In short, the more 'events' that this group of people are subjected to (including hospital admissions) generally leads to ↑ frailty, which is the biggest single predictor of mortality.

In addition, recurrent hospital admissions can contribute to the emergence of dependency and loss of confidence.

Bergman et al. (2007) described frailty as 'an adverse health state represented by an increased vulnerability to physical or psychological stressors because of decreased physiological reserve'.[2]

People living with type 2 diabetes (T2D) have a higher risk of developing frailty.[3]

It can be argued that it is an avoidable complication of diabetes and can be compounded by hypo- or hyperglycaemia.

It is essential that a frailty assessment is carried out at all health care opportunities—including as a routine part of the annual care processes (see ➲ Chapter 9). Checking a person's functional status and comorbidities with frailty, as opposed to age, should be used in determining the prognosis for older adults.

Make every contact count.

There are several frailty assessment tools, with some embedded into health care IT systems. When reviewing people for frailty, an approved tool,

eFI score	Category	Description
0–0.12	Fit	People who have no or few long-term conditions that are usually well controlled. This group would mainly be independent in day-to-day living activities
0.13–0.24	Mild frailty	People who are slowing up in older age and may need help with personal activities of daily living such as finances, shopping, transportation
0.25–0.36	Moderate frailty	People who have difficulties with outdoor activities and may have mobility problems or require help with activities such as washing and dressing
>0.36	Severe frailty	People who are often dependent for personal care and have a range of long-term conditions/multimorbidity. Some of this group may be medically stable but others can be unstable and at risk of dying within 6–12 months
eFI = electronic Frailty Index		

Fig. 13.1 Electronic Frailty Index.

Clinical Frailty Scale

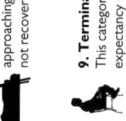

1 Very Fit – People who are robust, active, energetic and motivated. These people commonly exercise regularly. They are among the fittest for their age.

2 Well – People who have no active disease symptoms but are less fit than category 1. Often, they exercise or are very active occasionally, e.g. seasonally.

3 Managing Well – People whose medical problems are well controlled, but are not regularly active beyond routine walking.

4 Vulnerable – While not dependent on others for daily help, often symptoms limit activities. A common complaint is being "slowed up", and/or being tired during the day.

5 Mildly Frail – These people often have more evident slowing, and need help in high order IADLs (finances, transportation, heavy housework, medications). Typically, mild frailty progressively impairs shopping and walking outside alone, meal preparation and housework.

6 Moderately Frail – People need help with all outside activities and with keeping house. Inside, they often have problems with stairs and need help with bathing and might need minimal assistance (cuing, standby) with dressing.

7 Severely Frail – Completely dependent for personal care, from whatever cause (physical or cognitive). Even so, they seem stable and not at high risk of dying (within ~ 6 months).

8 Very Severely Frail – Completely dependent, approaching the end of life. Typically, they could not recover even from a minor illness.

9. Terminally Ill - Approaching the end of life. This category applies to people with a life expectancy <6 months, who are not otherwise evidently frail.

Scoring frailty in people with dementia

The degree of frailty corresponds to the degree of dementia. Common **symptoms in mild dementia** include forgetting the details of a recent event, though still remembering the event itself, repeating the same question/story and social withdrawal.

In **moderate dementia**, recent memory is very impaired, even though they seemingly can remember their past life events well. They can do personal care with prompting.

In **severe dementia**, they cannot do personal care without help.

Fig. 13.2 Rockwood Fraility Scale.

such as the ones illustrated in Figs 13.1 and 13.2, should be used and documented in the outcome of the assessment.

Frailty assessment scores include:
- Electronic Frailty Index (eFI)[4]
- Rockwood Scale[5]
- Timed Up and Go.[6]

People who are frail and have significant comorbidities or cognitive/functional impairment are unlikely to reap the benefits of intensification of treatments and are more likely to experience the side effects of over-intensification of therapies.[1]

Managing the older person with diabetes is complicated by:
- Other comorbidities
- Shortened life expectancy
- Potential adverse effects of treatment[1]
- Risk of falls due to loss of muscle mass and strength, other comorbidities, and general reduction in well-being
- Potential nutritional challenges.

References

1. Strain D, Down S, Brown P, Puttana A, Sinclair A. Diabetes and frailty: an expert consensus statement on the management of older adults with type 2 diabetes. *Diabetes Therapies.* 2021;**12**(5):1227–47.
2. Bergman H, Ferruci L, Guralnik J, *et al.* Frailty: An emerging research and clinical paradigm Issues and controversies. *Journals of Gerontology: Series A.* 2007;**62**(7):731–7.
3. Sinclair AJ; Task and Finish Group of Diabetes UK (2011). Good clinical practice guidelines for care home residents with diabetes: an executive summary. *Diabetic Medicine.* **28**(7):772–7.
4. NHS England. *Electronic Frailty Index.* Available at: ℘ www.england.nhs.uk/ourwork/clinical-policy/older-people/frailty/efi
5. Moorhouse P, Rockwood K. Rockwood Frailty Scale. Frailty, and its quantitative clinical evaluation. *Royal College of Physicians of Edinburgh.* 2012;**42**:333–40. Available at: ℘ www.england.nhs.uk/south/wp-content/uploads/sites/6/2022/02/rockwood-frailty-scale_.pdf
6. Mathias S, Nayak US, Isaacs B. Balance in elderly patients: the 'Get-Up and Go' test. *Archives of Physical Medicine and Rehabilitation.* 1986;**67**:387–9.

Individualizing targets

'*Targets*', including glycaemia, blood pressure, and lipids, should always be person-focused, by using guidance from evidence and evidence-based reviews.[1,2]

It is important that discussions around individualized targets are part of every assessment, opportunistic or planned.

The risks of hypoglycaemia not only on physical health (↑ risk of falls), but also on cognitive health and the recovery from these events, are significant.

For hypoglycaemia in older persons, there is blunting of the physiological adrenergic responses (tremor, sweating, palpitations), which may mean that blood glucose levels fall further before the onset of symptomatic hypoglycaemia.

Neuroglycopenic manifestations (confusion, sleepiness, aggression) may be mistaken for cognitive impairment (see ➜ Chapter 12).

For suggested glucose 'targets' in frailty see ➜ Chapter 7 Table 7.1.

References

1. Sinclair AJ; Task and Finish Group of Diabetes UK (2011). Good clinical practice guidelines for care home residents with diabetes: an executive summary. *Diabetic Medicine*. **28**(7):772–7.
2. Strain D, Hope S, Green A, Kar P, Valabji J, Sinclair A. Type 2 diabetes mellitus in older people: a brief statement of key principles of modern-day management including the assessment of frailty. *Diabetic Medication*. 2018;**35**(7):838–45.

Polypharmacy

Polypharmacy should always be at the top (or near the top) of the list of things to review, especially following a hospital admission.

Look to stop or suspend medication that is not needed or where the risk of side effects outweighs the benefits.

Deprescribing is as important as prescribing.

Also important is avoiding 'adding on' to current regimens without reviewing the effectiveness, contraindications, potential side effects, and concordance with current medication.[1]

When considering intensifying a regimen during an acute period of illness, consider the impact when the person returns home. Will the person require support with the additional medication or monitoring?

Make a clear plan for review of the regimen once the person is well again.

Simplify regimens as much as possible, ensuring that the person/family/carers understand the timing of medications.

Considerations in using glucose-lowering therapies include the following:
- Avoid the use of sulfonylurea and insulin therapies for frail people with T2D due to the risk of hypoglycaemia.
- If the above are used, ensure glucose monitoring is in place and educate the person/carers/family on hypoglycaemia (see ➲ Chapters 7 and 12).
- Review promptly following any hypoglycaemic event and reconsider the treatment plan.

Be aware of other risks, including:
- Renal impairment and need for dose adjustment (metformin, dipeptidyl peptidase type 4 (DPP-4) inhibitors); potential volume depletion with sodium–glucose cotransporter 2 (SGLT2) inhibitors
- Saxagliptin and pioglitazone—both contraindicated in heart failure
- Weight loss (can precipitate or exacerbate frailty)
- Fracture risk with pioglitazone in those with low bone density.

Ensuring nutritional health and minimizing weight loss

- Dietary intake should not be restricted but encouraged.
- Supplements or meal replacements often 'spike' the glucose level and are not always as enjoyable as something that the person would prefer to eat.
- Optimizing nutrition and how to achieve this should be discussed with the person or their advocate.
- There is still conflicting advice around diabetes and what people are 'allowed' to eat. Look to dispel any such 'myths'.
- Include engagement with the nutrition team.

Multidisciplinary teamworking

Consider support from all appropriate multidisciplinary team (MDT) members, including physiotherapists, dietitians, and social prescribing.

Reference

1. Sinclair A, Gallagher A (2019). *Managing frailty and associated comorbidities in older adults with diabetes: Position Statement on behalf of the Association of British Clinical Diabetologists (ABCD)*. Available at: ℘ https://abcd.care/resource/managing-frailty-and-associated-comorbidities-older-adults-diabetes-position-statement

Nursing and care homes

People with diabetes, who are living in a care or nursing home, are by de-fault vulnerable and frail, and rely on others to either co-manage or fully manage their diabetes.

The risk of hypoglycaemia, hyperglycaemia, and foot problems are ↑ if people are unable to monitor their own glucose levels or carry out daily foot checks.

This can be compounded if access to diabetes education and diabetes experience are limited amongst care home staff.

The National Advisory Panel on Care Home Diabetes (2022) found that shortfalls in diabetes care are associated with suboptimal treatment, poor clinical outcomes, poor quality of life, and reduced survival.[1]

All people working in community teams or nursing/care homes should have a basic understanding of diabetes care, including acknowledgement of the complexity that living with diabetes can involve extending to ethical principles and the importance of emotional well-being.

Appropriate assessment and care planning are key to a person's needs being met.

Reference

1. National Advisory Panel on Care Home Diabetes (2022). *A strategic document of diabetes care for care homes.* Available at: ℘ http://fdrop.net/wp-content/uploads/2022/05/FINAL-NAPCHD-Main-document-for-FDROP-website-08-05-22.pdf

Further reading

Sinclair AJ, Bellary S, Middleton A, *et al.* Type 1 Diabetes in care homes: A practical guide on man-agement. *Diabetic Medicine.* 2024 Nov 5:e15457. doi:10.1111/dme.15457. Epub ahead of print. PMID: 39500566.

End of life

Individuals are 'approaching the end of life' when they are likely to die within the next 12 months. These include individuals whose death is imminent (expected within a few hours or days) and those with general frailty and coexisting conditions.[1]

Priorities are to:
- Keep the person safe
- Avoid osmotic symptoms
- Avoid hypoglycaemia
- Avoid diabetic ketoacidosis (DKA)
- Avoid hyperosmolar hyperglycaemic state (HHS).

Guidelines suggest that glucose levels should be 'no less than 6mmol and no more than 15mmol' (TREND, 2024).[2] This can, however, be individualized following the end-of-life planning review.

Key 'take-home' messages

Involve the person with diabetes, their family members and carers, and other health care professionals, so that an appropriate plan of care is place.

- Consider what is 'normal' for the person, along with current guidelines around therapeutic targets.
- A holistic, individualized approach is key.
- Proactive risk identification—assess the functional status and degree of frailty.
- Focus on person-related safety, polypharmacy, and medication side effects, as well as deprescribing.
- Anticipatory care planning with admission avoidance.
- Consider medical comorbidities.
- Consider life expectancy.
- Care from across the whole MDT.
- Maintain quality of life.

It is not uncommon for people with diabetes to require hospital admission either because of their diabetes or with their diabetes. During admission, especially if there is an acute illness, full optimization of glucose levels, including starting insulin or intensifying medication, may take place. On discharge, when considering transfer of care, particularly from secondary to community or primary, it is important to review a person's pre-admission status and management of their diabetes to ensure the levels of intensity can be maintained post-discharge.

When handing over insulin therapy to a third person (particularly community nursing teams), consider the regimen in line with what the person can manage and what community nursing teams can support them with. For example, a multiple daily injection (MDI) regimen is not the ideal choice for a person relying on community nursing teams—primarily because of the timing of the insulin, but also because of the capacity of community nurses. Unrealistic treatment plans can put significant burdens on resources.

References

1. Sinclair AJ; Task and Finish Group of Diabetes UK (2011). Good clinical practice guidelines for care home residents with diabetes: an executive summary. *Diabetic Medicine*. **28**(7):772–7.
2. TREND Diabetes (2024). *End of life guidance for diabetes care*. Available at: ℅ https://trenddiabetes.online/wp-content/uploads/2024/06/EoL_TREND_2024_v11-1.pdf

Case study

Mrs M aged 81 yrs

Lives in a care home and the district nurse visits weekly for catheter care.

Has severe frailty (Level 7 on Rockwood Frailty Score)

Known T2D for 12 years, usually taking Metformin 500mgs twice daily and a DPP4 inhibitor daily.

Most recent HbA1c is 68mmol/mol (previous range 63–70mmol/mol)

Does not self-monitor glucose levels unless the care home staff are requested to do so.

Admitted to hospital with a urinary tract infection and high glucose levels (mid-teens)

Oral medication stopped in hospital due to acute kidney injury (lowered eGFR) and commenced on basal bolus insulin regime

On discharge, insulin being administered by community nurses as care home staff not trained to administer insulin.

Community diabetes team asked to review Mrs M as multiple episodes of Mrs M being 'unsteady' and some 'dizziness'.

- A continuous glucose monitor was used to assess glucose levels.
- The glucose data showed a significant risk of hypoglycaemia, to include overnight when the carers may not have been monitoring capillary glucose levels (see CGM data)
- The short-term use of CGM helped demonstrate that an intensive MDI regimen was not necessary for this lady now her acute illness had resolved.
- Mrs M was subsequently transferred back to her pre-admission diabetes medication after a repeat blood test showed that her eGFR levels had recovered following the urinary tract infection.

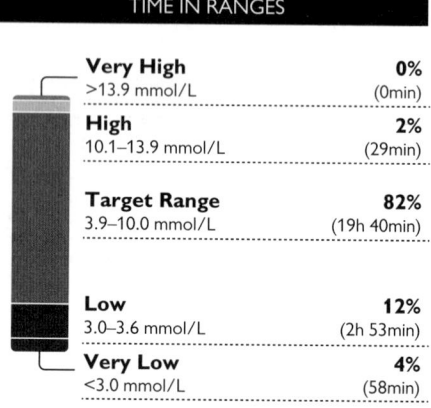

TIME IN RANGES		
Very High >13.9 mmol/L	**0%** (0min)	
High 10.1–13.9 mmol/L	**2%** (29min)	
Target Range 3.9–10.0 mmol/L	**82%** (19h 40min)	
Low 3.0–3.6 mmol/L	**12%** (2h 53min)	
Very Low <3.0 mmol/L	**4%** (58min)	

Chapter 14

Female health and diabetes

Female sexual dysfunction

Sexual dysfunction among women living with diabetes is twice as common, compared with women without diabetes. A recent meta-analysis and systematic review highlighted a prevalence of 58.81% in all diabetes with women with type 2 diabetes (T2D) more likely to experience sexual dysfunction with a prevalence of 71.03%.[1]

Reasons for a higher prevalence in diabetes include:[2]

- Low or high glucose levels causing possible:
  - Lack of vaginal lubrication
  - Subsequent pain during sexual activity (dyspareunia)
  - Structural changes in female genital tissue plus impairment of nerve and blood supply, which might impact the arousal and orgasmic sexual response
- Higher rates of depression and diabetes-related distress, which can lead to low sexual drive
- Wearing of diabetes devices, such as insulin pumps and continuous glucose monitors, which may affect body image and self-esteem
- Lumps from lipohypertrophy around insulin injection sites, which may also affect body image and self-esteem
- The burden of self-managing diabetes, which may affect the spontaneity of sex.

Untreated sexual dysfunction can lead to relationship difficulties and breakdown.

There is also evidence that women with diabetes and sexual dysfunction can experience cardiovascular and neurological complications.[3]

The area of female sexual dysfunction (FSD) is under-researched and there are still gaps in our knowledge as to how best to support women experiencing difficulties. However, raising awareness of the problem may help women living with diabetes and health care professionals (HCPs) to discuss it as part of routine diabetes clinical consultations.

It is reported that:

- 72% of women with FSD would like to talk to their HCP about their difficulties
- 73% of these women would like their HCP to initiate the conversation.[2]

Self-report questionnaires or clinician checklists may assist women and HCPs in identifying specific problems. For example, the 19-item Female Sexual Function Index (FSFI)[4] or the Decreased Sexual Desire Screener[5] could be incorporated into diabetes consultations.

Management

This may include:

- Optimization of lifestyle factors where appropriate (e.g. smoking cessation, weight loss)
- Optimization of glycaemia
- Use of gels and lubrication for any vaginal dryness
- Psychological interventions (see ➲ Chapter 8)
- Pharmacotherapy treatments for sexual dysfunction in women with diabetes such as phosphodiesterase 5 (PDE5) inhibitors—have

demonstrated improvements in sexual arousal, for example, but most studies have limitations such as using non-validated questionnaires to measure outcome, small sample sizes, and lack of an appropriate control group.[2]

References

1. Gebeyehu NA, Gesese MM, Tegegne KD, *et al*. Global prevalence of sexual dysfunction among diabetic patients from 2008 to 2022: systematic review and meta-analysis. *Metabolism Open*. 2023;**18**:100247.
2. Winkley K, Kristensen C, Fosbury J. Sexual health and function in women with diabetes. *Diabetic Medicine*. 2021;**38**:e14644.
3. Kingsberg SA, Schaffir J, Faught BM, *et al*. Female sexual health: barriers to optimal outcomes and a roadmap for improved patient–clinician communications. *Journal of Women's Health (Larchmont)*. 2019;**28**(4):432–43.
4. Rosen CBJHSLR. The Female Sexual Function Index (FSFI): a multidimensional self-report instrument for the assessment of female sexual function. *Journal of Sex & Marital Therapy*. 2000;**26**(2).
5. Clayton AH, Goldstein I, Kim NN, *et al*. The International Society for the Study of Women's Sexual Health Process of Care for Management of Hypoactive Sexual Desire Disorder in Women. *Mayo Clinic Proceedings*. 2018;**93**(4):467–87.

Polycystic ovary syndrome

Polycystic ovary syndrome (PCOS) is an endocrine condition which can affect 6–15% of women of reproductive age. It is associated with insulin resistance and hyperinsulinaemia, thus increasing the risk of development of T2D and/or cardiovascular disease (CVD).

PCOS may be treated with weight optimization through diet and ↑ physical activity. Pharmacological treatment is commonly with metformin.

Any women with PCOS should be supported with lifestyle optimization and screened regularly for T2D.[1]

Reference

Livadas S, Anagnostis P, Bosdou JK, *et al.* Polycystic ovary syndrome and type 2 diabetes mellitus: A state-of-the-art review. *World J Diabetes.* 2022 Jan 15;**13**(1):5–26. doi:10.4239/wjd.v13.i1.5. PMID: 35070056; PMCID: PMC8771268.

Preconception care

Whilst the rates of unintended pregnancy have ↓ in recent years, nearly half of pregnancies are still unplanned. In women with pre-existing diabetes, appropriate pre-pregnancy planning is one of the most important steps in reducing the risk of birth defects, as these can take place very early in pregnancy.

Babies of women with diabetes are five times as likely to be stillborn and twice as likely to have a major congenital anomaly, when compared with the general maternity population.

Women with diabetes also have significantly higher rates of miscarriage, pre-eclampsia, perinatal mortality, preterm delivery, and macrosomia, when compared with the background population. Suboptimal glycaemic levels, both before and in the early stages of pregnancy, are associated with adverse pregnancy outcomes.

To reduce the risk of adverse outcomes for both mother and baby, it is recommended that women with pre-existing diabetes achieve an HbA1c of ≤48mmol/mol prior to conception. To achieve this, women with type 1 diabetes (T1D) should be offered a hybrid closed-loop system (see ➲ Chapter 6). Women with early-onset T2D should be referred to specialist preconception services, where available, to optimize their glucose management.

Many oral and non-insulin injectable therapies for glucose lowering are not licensed for use during pregnancy.

The National Pregnancy in Diabetes Audit (NPDA)[1] identified that only 9.5% of women with T2D were well prepared for pregnancy, compared with 17.6% of women with T1D. Rates were even lower in women living in more socio-economically deprived areas and in women from ethnic minorities.

Preparation for pregnancy can be time-consuming and take several months to achieve the desired HbA1c, and therefore, knowledge of local services for preconception care and early referral are important.

Early referral allows for specialist advice, including full cardiorenal and retinal assessment, reinforcing the importance of smoking and alcohol cessation, medication safety and review, supporting the achievement of HbA1c levels below 48mmol/mol prior to pregnancy, and ensuring folic acid 5mg is prescribed daily for at least 3 months prior to, and for the first 12 weeks of, pregnancy.[2]

It is advisable to offer contraceptive advice if glucose levels are not optimal for conception, especially if HbA1c is >86mmol/mol, where pregnancy is strongly advised against.

Contraception

The full range of contraceptive methods is normally suitable for women with diabetes, but use of combined oral contraception for the woman who is normotensive, whose diabetes management is stable, and who has no signs of complications should be accompanied by regular diabetes review and surveillance. Long-acting reversible contraception (LARC) may be an appropriate contraception of choice for women living with diabetes.

Ensure provision of up-to-date information on the full range of contraceptive methods available, clinics in the locality, and access to relevant and appropriate websites and useful literature.

Allow plenty of time for discussion and ensure an appropriate environment to maintain confidentiality and encourage a relaxed conversation.

Remember that to be effective, the chosen contraception must be used properly, and therefore acceptable to the woman and ideally her partner.

For up-to-date criteria for contraceptive advice, please see the link to the UK a Eligibility Criteria (UKMEC) for contraceptive use (available at: ℘ www.fsrh.org/standards-and-guidance/fsrh-guidelines-and-statements/contraception-for-specific-populations/).

Women who wish to become pregnant should have the following care

- Referral as soon as possible to a preconception diabetes clinic or to the specialist diabetes care team. A referral 1–2 years prior to planned conception may be appropriate.
- Prescribe folic acid 5mg daily for at least 3 months prior to conception and until the woman is 12 weeks pregnant, to minimize the risk of a neural tube defect.
- Offer smoking and alcohol cessation advice, as appropriate.
- Check HbA1c monthly.
- Review current medications:
  - Discontinue angiotensin-converting enzyme inhibitors and commence an alternative treatment for throughout the pregnancy if indicated, for example: labetalol, nifedipine, methyldopa.
  - Discontinue statins at least 3 months prior to conception and for the entire pregnancy.
  - If on oral hypoglycaemic agents other than metformin, look to conversion to insulin under supervision of the diabetes care team and provide continuous glucose monitoring.
  - Discontinue sodium–glucose cotransporter 2 (SGLT2) inhibitors prior to conception.
  - Discontinue glucagon-like peptide 1 receptor agonist (GLP1-RA) therapy at least 3 months prior to conception.
  - Continue contraception until advised otherwise by the specialist team or HbA1c is <48mmol/mol.
- Offer continuous glucose monitoring to women with T2D on insulin therapy.
- Offer hybrid closed loop or continuous glucose monitoring and insulin pump therapy to women with T1D.
- Provide lifestyle advice and support, including, where relevant, support with optimizing weight.
- Ensure regular attendance at retinal screening.
- Ensure regular urine albumin:creatinine ratio (ACR) testing.
- Ensure adequate supplies of both glucose and in T1D, ketone monitoring equipment are made available, in addition to any continuous glucose monitoring.

NB in women of childbearing potential who are living with overweight or obesity, GLP1-RA (with or without glucose-dependent insulinotropic polypeptide [GIP-1]) therapy may be used to optimize glucose levels, with the benefit of weight loss. This would be used 1–2 years before desired conception. The incretin therpay would need to be stopped at least 3 months prior to pregnancy. Robust contraception must be used when taking the GLP1-RA (with or without GIP-1), particularly because any weight loss could ↑ fertility.

References

1. NHS England (2023). *National Pregnancy in Diabetes Audit 2021–2022*. Available at: ℘ https://digital.nhs.uk/data-and-information/publications/statistical/national-pregnancy-in-diabetes-audit
2. National Institute for Health and Care Excellence (2015, last updated 2020). *Diabetes in pregnancy: management from preconception to the postnatal period*. NICE guideline [NG3]. Available at: ℘ www.nice.org.uk/guidance/ng3

Further reading

NHS England (2023). *Saving babies lives version three: a care bundle for reducing perinatal mortality*. Available at: ℘ www.england.nhs.uk/wp-content/uploads/2023/05/PRN00614-Saving-babies-lives-version-three-a-care-bundle-for-reducing-perinatal-mortality.pdf
TREND (2024). Planning for a baby when you have diabetes Available at: ℘ https://trenddiabetes.online/portfolio/planning-for-a-baby-when-you-have-diabetes/

Menopause and diabetes

Diabetes and menopause are both cardiometabolic conditions. Low oestrogen levels can affect insulin production and increase central adiposity, insulin resistance, and the risk of developing T2D.

It can have a significant impact on glucose variability, thus making management of glucose levels challenging in both T1D and T2D.

Many of the symptoms of the menopause, hypo- and hyperglycaemia, and diabetes neuropathies overlap.

Symptoms of the menopause include:
- Anxiety
- Low mood
- Fatigue
- Headaches/migraines
- Dizziness
- Sleep disturbance
- Body temperature changes
- Muscle aches and joint pains
- Cognitive changes
- Genitourinary problems
- Loss of libido
- Skin and hair changes
- Dry eyes
- Tinnitus
- Gastrointestinal changes.

The Menopause Symptom Questionnaire is a useful tool in assessing for symptoms (available at: ℜ www.themenopausecharity.org/2021/10/21/menopause-symptoms-questionnaire).

Management Considerations Include:
- Hormonal replacement therapy (HRT) can be considered for all women experiencing symptoms associated with the perimenopause and menopause.
- For most women, HRT benefits outweigh its risks.
- HRT has been shown to have cardiometabolic benefits.
- Incorporate normal strategies for reduction in cardiovascular risk and the risk of osteoporosis.
- Transdermal oestrogen does not carry an ↑ risk of venous thromboembolism and may be considered for those with diabetes, hypertension, obesity, and CVD. It is important to seek specialised advice as required.
- HRT generally improves mental and physical well-being, which can lead to positive health outcomes.
- It is always important to ask about genitourinary health and to use vaginal hormonal therapy, alone or in conjunction with HRT, as needed.
- Women taking diabetes medications that can cause hypoglycaemia should have access to blood glucose monitoring and reduce/adjust their medications based on blood glucose levels.
- Support optimization of lifestyle where appropriate—for example, smoking cessation, weight optimization, and reduction in cardiovascular risk factors (e.g. hypertension, dyslipidaemia) (see ➲ Chapter 10).

Further reading

Hillard T, Abernethy K, Hamoda H. *Management of the Menopause*, 6th edition. Marlow: British Menopause Society, 2017.

Paschou SA, Anagnostis P, Pavlou DI, Vryonidou A, Goulis DG, Lambrinoudaki I. Diabetes in menopause: risks and management. *Current Vascular Pharmacology*. 2019;**17**(6):556–63.

NICE NG23 (2015 and updated 2024). Menopause: identification and management. Available at: ✑ https://www.nice.org.uk/guidance/ng23

TREND (2021). Diabetes and the Menopause. Available at: ✑ https://trenddiabetes.online/portfolio/diabetes-and-the-menopause/

Chapter 15

Diabetes in pregnancy

Introduction

The classification of diabetes during pregnancy falls into two categories:
- Pre-existing diabetes
- Gestational diabetes mellitus (GDM).

Pre-existing diabetes would usually be T1D or T2D but could also include maturity-onset diabetes of the young (MODY), slowly evolving immune-mediated diabetes, chemical/drug-induced diabetes, pancreatitis-related diabetes, and cystic fibrosis. The latest National Pregnancy in Diabetes (NPID) audit data[1] show a changing demographic in pre-existing diabetes, with more pregnant women with T2D (55%) compared with those with T1D (44%). The NPID also identified that only 9.5% of women with T2D were well prepared for pregnancy, compared with 17.6% of women with T1D. Rates were even lower in women living in more socio-economic-deprived areas and in women from ethnic minorities.

GDM is defined as a carbohydrate intolerance which results in raised blood glucose levels (hyperglycaemia) that is first identified in pregnancy.[2]

References

1. NHS England (2021/2022). *National Pregnancy in Diabetes Audit (2021/2022)*. Available at: ℜ https://digital.nhs.uk/data-and-information/publications/statistical/national-pregnancy-in-diabetes-audit
2. National Institute for Health and Care Excellence (2015, updated 2020). *Diabetes in pregnancy: management from preconception to the postpartum period*. NICE guideline [NG3]. Available at: ℜ www.nice.org.uk/guidance/ng3

Managing diabetes in pregnancy

Diabetes and obstetric specialist teams aim to support women to monitor and manage their glucose levels effectively and safely throughout their pregnancy and for a short time postnatally.

Suboptimal glucose levels during pregnancy can lead to complications such as:[1]
- Miscarriage
- Pre-eclampsia
- Fetal macrosomia (fetus larger than average for gestational age)
- Polyhydramnios (excessive amniotic fluid surrounding the fetus)
- Preterm birth/induction of labour and/or caesarean section
- Trauma during birth/shoulder dystocia
- Neonatal hypoglycaemia
- Neonatal admission
- Perinatal death
- Fetal malformations.

Barriers to achieving optimal glucose levels may include:
- Lack of understanding of the importance of good glucose management
- Difficulties maintaining the demanding regimen of glucose monitoring and frequent medication adjustments
- Mental health challenges such as anxiety and stress
- Health and cultural beliefs.

Difficulties in managing glucose levels in pregnancy are also related to carbohydrate metabolism and insulin resistance.

Throughout pregnancy and after birth, insulin requirements change markedly (see Fig. 15.1).[2] This is driven by the action of pregnancy hormones.

In late pregnancy, there is more day-to-day variability related to increasingly delayed insulin absorption.[3]

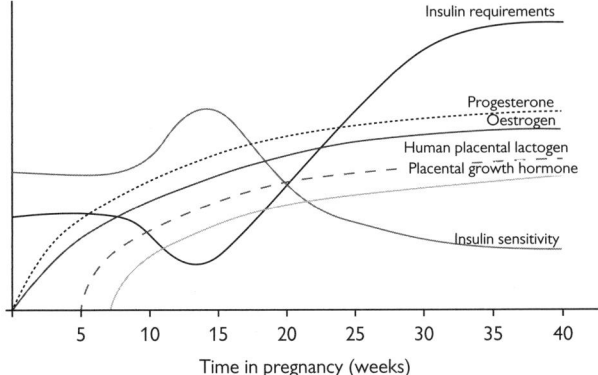

Fig. 15.1 Normal pregnancy hormones and insulin resistance.
Lam et al., 2021[4]

References

1. National Institute for Health and Care Excellence (2015, updated 2020). *Diabetes in pregnancy: management from preconception to the postpartum period*. NICE guideline [NG3]. Available at: ℘ www.nice.org.uk/guidance/ng3
2. ABCD DTN-UK (2020). *Best practice guide: using diabetes technology in pregnancy*. Version 2.0. Available at: ℘ https://abcd.care/sites/default/files/site_uploads/Resources/DTN/BP-Pregnancy-DTN-V2.0.pdf
3. Goudie RJB, Lunn D, Hovorka R, Murphy HR. Pharmacokinetics of insulin aspart in pregnant women with type 1 diabetes: Every day is different. *Diabetes Care*. 2014;**37**(6):e121–e122.
4. Lam AYR, Lim W, McMicking J, *et al.* (2021). Clinical management of diabetes in pregnancy. *The Global Library of Women's Medicine*. ℘ https://doi.org/10.3843/GLOWM.416423

Gestational diabetes mellitus

Identifying risk

Assess the following risk factors in all pregnant women at their booking appointment:[1]

- BMI above 30kg/m²
- Previous macrosomic baby >4.5kg
- Previous GDM
- Family history of diabetes (first-degree relative)
- Ethnicity with a high prevalence of diabetes.

Consider further testing to exclude GDM if:

- Glycosuria 2+ on one occasion, or
- Glycosuria 1+ on two occasions.

If one of the above risk factors is identified, then a 75g 2-hour oral glucose tolerance test (OGTT) should be offered at 24–28 weeks' gestation.

If the risk factor is identified of a woman having had GDM in a previous pregnancy, offer as soon as possible after booking either:

- Early self-monitoring of glucose levels, or
- Early OGTT (if this is normal, then repeat OGTT at 24–28 weeks' gestation).

It is also recommended that if GDM is diagnosed early, HbA1c is obtained to identify possible undiagnosed T2D.

Diagnosis and management of gestational diabetes mellitus[1]

- Fasting plasma glucose level of 5.6mmol/L or above, or
- 2-hour plasma glucose level of >7.8mmol/L or above.

If diagnosed with GDM, then offer a review in a multidisciplinary diabetes/antenatal clinic within 1 week. This should include a diabetologist, an obstetrician, a diabetes specialist midwife (DSM), a diabetes specialist nurse (DSN), and a dietitian.

Women should be referred to a dietitian for dietary advice. The important role exercise can play in managing glucose levels should also be discussed.

Women will be required to self-monitor their glucose levels. The aim would be to maintain glucose levels at:[1]

- <5.3mmol fasting and/or pre-meal
- <7.8mmol 1-hour post-meal.

If the above glucose targets are not met with dietary changes and ↑ activity levels within 1–2 weeks, then metformin should be considered.

Insulin therapy should be offered if glucose targets are not achieved with metformin.

Insulin and metformin should be offered immediately after a diagnosis of GDM if:

- Fasting OGTT is 7mmol/L or above, or
- Fasting OGTT is 6.0–6.9mmol/L and macrosomia or polyhydramnios is present.

If insulin is commenced, there should be a discussion about the risks of hypoglycaemia and the importance of having fast-acting glucose available if needed (see ⟴ Chapter 12).

Glucose levels should be reviewed every 1–2 weeks by the diabetes team either remotely or in face-to-face clinic.

There is a requirement that women inform the Driver and Vehicle Licensing Agency (DVLA) if insulin treatment lasts (or will last) for over 3 months. Glucose levels need to be >5mmol to be safe to drive, and they need to be rechecked every 2 hours if driving for longer periods or several shorter journeys.[2]

Monitoring of the fetus

Ultrasound scans will be offered, in addition to the 12- to 13-week scan, at:
- 20 weeks' gestation to detect any structural abnormalities
- 28 weeks' gestation (every 4 weeks thereafter) to measure fetal growth and amniotic fluid volume.

There may be a more individualized approach if there are any pregnancy complications.

Await spontaneous labour but advise that timing of delivery for women with GDM would usually be before 40+6 weeks' gestation, so induction of labour or caesarean section may be offered.[1]

References

1. National Institute for Health and Care Excellence (2015, updated 2020). *Diabetes in pregnancy: management from preconception to the postpartum period*. NICE guideline [NG3]. Available at: ℗ www.nice.org.uk/guidance/ng3
2. Driver and Vehicle Licensing Agency (2016, updated 2024). *Assessing fitness to drive: a guide for medical professionals*. Available at: ℗ www.gov.uk/government/publications/assessing-fitness-to-drive-a-guide-for-medical-professionals

Management of pre-existing diabetes in pregnancy

The National Institute for Health and Care Excellence (NICE)[1] recommends that pregnancies are planned (see ➲ Chapter 14). Women should receive support during this time to manage their diabetes, to include retinal screening and renal assessment.

Once the pregnancy is confirmed, a booking appointment should ideally be scheduled before 10 weeks' gestation. The NPID audit highlighted that unfortunately the majority of women with T2D did not present to specialist diabetes antenatal clinics until over 14 weeks' gestation, compared with the majority of women with T1D who presented at around 5–6 weeks' gestation.

Referral for retinal screening should be completed as soon as possible after confirming the pregnancy, especially if the last retinal screening has not been within the last 3 months. First- and third-trimester screening should take place, with an additional screening in the second trimester if there is retinopathy present.

Bloods and renal assessment should be carried out at the first contact with the diabetes/antenatal team after pregnancy is confirmed.

NB women who need treatment for retinopathy and/or renal impairment may need to be managed in a maternal medicine clinic (MMC) or a multidisciplinary team (MDT) clinic with an MMC plan.[3]

NHS guidance on diabetes in pregnancy[3] recommends 5mg of folic acid in the preconception period and for the first 12 weeks of pregnancy. This helps to prevent babies from developing neural tube defects such as spina bifida.

Women who have pre-existing diabetes should have immediate contact with the joint diabetes and antenatal clinic when they discover they are pregnant and 1- to 2-weekly contact throughout the pregnancy.[1]

The importance of 'joined-up support' in a 'one-stop clinic' was highlighted in Saving Babies' Lives[2] in order to reduce pregnancy complications.

Remote consultations are useful for supporting women in between face-to-face appointments.[4]

A viability ultrasound scan should be scheduled at 7–9 weeks' gestation.

Low-dose aspirin 150mg once a day from 12 weeks' gestation is recommended for women with a high risk of pre-eclampsia, including women with pre-existing diabetes, and will be continued to the 36th week of pregnancy.[3]

Women are aiming for HbA1c at conception of 48mmol/mol or lower. HbA1c will be checked at the booking appointment to determine the level of risk for the pregnancy and may be considered in the second and third trimesters.

For routine assessment of glycaemic management during pregnancy, capillary blood glucose monitoring (CBGM) or continuous glucose monitoring (CGM) data will be used.

Glucose targets for women with pre-existing diabetes

Targets are the same as those in GDM if using fingerstick blood glucose.

If using a continuous glucose sensor, targets for women with T1D are:

- 3.5–7.8mmol/L at least 70% of the time
- >7.8mmol/L <25% of the time
- <3.5mmol/L <4% of the time
- <3.0mmol/L <1% of the time.

There is limited evidence and, at the time of writing no current consensus guidelines, to support the time-in-range targets for women with T2D using CGM during pregnancy.

For some women with early-onset T2D (EOT2D), >70% time in range may be suitable, but >90% may be a more appropriate target in many women with EOT2D, especially if recently diagnosed and/or with HbA1c <48mmol/mol (6.5%) prior to pregnancy.[5]

The challenges are that the risk of hypoglycaemia must be balanced against the risk of hyperglycaemia to the fetus.[4]

As with GDM, any women who are on insulin should always have access to fast-acting glucose to prevent and treat hypoglycaemia. Women with T1D should also have glucagon via an injection available, and relatives should be instructed on how to administer this if needed. Impaired awareness of hypoglycaemia, particularly in the first trimester, should be discussed.

Women with T1D should also be offered a ketone meter and strips, with advice regarding sick day guidance in pregnancy.

It is recommended that testing for ketonaemia for any woman with diabetes is performed if they are hyperglycaemic or unwell.[1]

Fetal monitoring in relation to ultrasound scans follows a similar schedule to that for women with GDM.

Perinatal mortality

Maternity services in England and Wales that provide care to pregnant women with pre-existing diabetes submit annual data to NPID.[6] These data are used to address challenges and develop action plans.

Data from NPID (2021/22) showed that in pregnant women with diabetes, the risk of experiencing a stillbirth is 4–5 times higher than that in the background population.

A care bundle for reducing perinatal mortality, with an additional element added relating to pre-existing diabetes in pregnancy, was published in July 2023.[3] This guidance is currently being implemented by NHS trusts that manage women with pre-existing diabetes who are pregnant.

The guidance includes:
- Using HbA1c to risk-stratify and provide additional support
- An MDT pathway approach to management of pregnancies
- Clear documentation of assessing glucose digitally
- Offering consistent access to CGM
- CGM training for the MDT and expertise to support CGM and other technologies
- Guidance in managing women with DKA.

Pregnancy is a ketogenic state and women who are pregnant have a higher risk of developing DKA.[4] This can occur when glucose levels are considered 'normal'.[7] This risk of DKA is higher for women on continuous subcutaneous insulin infusion (CSII), so it is important to ensure that they have 'backup' insulin pens to be used if the insulin pump fails.[4]

DKA in pregnancy carries a risk of fetal death of 16–27% or higher.[8] Women who are admitted to hospital in DKA should have ongoing multi-disciplinary consultant input.[3]

References

1. National Institute for Health and Care Excellence (2015, updated 2020). *Diabetes in pregnancy: management from preconception to the postpartum period*. NICE guideline [NG3]. Available at: 🔗 www.nice.org.uk/guidance/ng3
2. NHS England (2024). *Diabetes and pregnancy*. Available at: 🔗 www.nhs.uk/pregnancy/related-conditions/existing-health-conditions/diabetes
3. NHS England (2023). *Saving Babies' Lives, version 3. A care bundle for reducing perinatal mortality*. Available at: 🔗 www.england.nhs.uk/long-read/saving-babies-lives-version-3
4. ABCD DTN-UK (2020). *Best practice guide: using diabetes technology in pregnancy*. Version 2.0. Available at: 🔗 https://abcd.care/sites/default/files/site_uploads/Resources/DTN/BP-Pregnancy-DTN-V2.0.pdf
5. Battelino T, Danne T, Bergenstal RM, *et al*. Clinical targets for continuous glucose monitoring data interpretation: recommendations from the international consensus on time in range. *Diabetes Care*. 2019;**42**(8):1593–603.
6. NHS England (2021/2022). *National Pregnancy in Diabetes Audit (2021/2022)*. Available at: 🔗 https://digital.nhs.uk/data-and-information/publications/statistical/national-pregnancy-in-diabetes-audit
7. Joint British Diabetes Societies for Inpatient Care (2023). *Managing diabetes and hyperglycaemia during labour and birth*. Available at: 🔗 https://abcd.care/sites/default/files/site_uploads/JBDS_Guidelines_Current/JBDS_12_Managing_diabetes_and_hyperglycaemia_during_labour_and_birth_with_QR_code_February_2023.pdf
8. Morrison FJR, Movassaghian M, Seely EW, *et al*. (2017). Fetal outcomes after diabetic ketoacidosis during pregnancy. *Diabetes Care*. **40**(7):e77–379.

Diabetes technology in pregnancy

Diabetes technology, including CGM, CSII, and hybrid closed loop (HCL), has been shown to provide benefit in pregnancy[1,2] (see ➲ Chapter 6).

Real-time CGM should be offered to all women with T1D who are pregnant. Feig et al.[2] highlighted that women who started CGM in the first trimester vs CBGM improved their glycaemic management and improved neonatal outcomes. Women who have pre-existing diabetes who are on multiple-dose insulin (MDI) should be offered CGM[3] if they are having difficulties with achieving pregnancy glucose targets despite efforts or are experiencing significant disabling hypoglycaemia.

HCL should be offered to all women with T1D who are planning a pregnancy or are pregnant.[4]

Smart insulin pens, also known as connected pens, can also be used in pregnant women with diabetes if information is needed about the timing and amount of insulin given. They show how much insulin was given at the time of the last dose. They can be paired with some mobile phone applications which allow data from CGM and a smart pen to be stored in one place.

References

1. Lee TTM, Collett C, Man MS, et al.; AiDAPT Collaborative Group. AiDAPT: automated insulin delivery in women with pregnancy complicated by type 1 diabetes. *New England Journal of Medicine*. 2023;**389**:1566–78. doi: 10.1056/NEJMoa2303911.

2. Feig DS, Donovan LE, Corcoy R, et al. Continuous glucose monitoring in pregnant women with type 1 diabetes (CONCEPTT): a multicentre international randomised controlled trial. *The Lancet*. 2017;**390**(10110):2347–59. doi: 10.1016/S0140-6736(17)32400-5.

3. National Institute for Health and Care Excellence (2015, updated 2020). *Diabetes in pregnancy: management from preconception to the postpartum period*. NICE guideline [NG3]. Available at: ⊕ www.nice.org.uk/guidance/ng3

4. National Institute for Health and Care Excellence (2023). *Hybrid closed loop systems for managing blood glucose levels in type 1 diabetes*. Technology appraisal guidance [TA943]. Available at: ⊕ www.nice.org.uk/guidance/ta943/chapter/1-Recommendations

Supporting mental health

The psychological impact and time commitment required to manage diabetes in pregnancy for women should not be underestimated.[1]

People with diabetes are more than twice as likely to be diagnosed with depression.[2]

The extra information that CGM offers can be overwhelming and the psychological impact of seeing 'out-of-range' glucose can be difficult to cope with.[1]

The role of the MDT in providing support to all women with diabetes in relation to their mental health is crucial (see ➲ Chapter 8).

Strategies include:

- Referral to specialist mental health midwifery teams, if available.
- Psychological support within diabetes teams
- Improving Access to Psychological Therapies (IAPT) referral.
- Encouraging women to access other support networks they may find helpful.

References

1. ABCD DTN-UK (2020). *Best practice guide: using diabetes technology in pregnancy*. Version 2.0. Available at: ℜ https://abcd.care/sites/default/files/site_uploads/Resources/DTN/BP-Pregnancy-DTN-V2.0.pdf
2. Diabetes UK (2019). *Diabetes and emotional health. A practical guide for healthcare professionals supporting adults with type 1 and type 2 diabetes*. Available at: ℜ www.diabetes.org.uk/resources-s3/2019-03/0506%20Diabetes%20UK%20Australian%20Handbook_P4_FINAL_1.pdf

Safeguarding

Diabetes and obstetric specialist teams may also be required to support women in relation to specific safeguarding concerns:

- Domestic abuse is more likely to begin or escalate during pregnancy. This can have negative health implications for pregnant women and their babies; >40% of survivors experience mental health issues, including anxiety and depression.[1]
- Women who are the most socio-economically deprived and particularly those from South Asian and Black ethnicities have a higher risk of perinatal mortality.[2]
- Support for women may involve liaising with social services. This may include basic needs such as clothing/food availability/cooking facilities.

Saving Babies' Lives[3] highlights that some women may also need asylum support.

References

1. Saving Babies' Lives Version 3: A Care Bundle for reducing perinatal mortality. (June 2023). Available at: ℜ https://www.england.nhs.uk/long-read/saving-babies-lives-version-3/
2. NHS England (2024). *Diabetes and pregnancy*. Available at: ℜ www.nhs.uk/pregnancy/related-conditions/existing-health-conditions/diabetes

Diabetes and intrapartum care for women with diabetes in pregnancy

Women with pre-existing diabetes may be offered induction of labour or a caesarean section.

Timing of delivery for women with pre-existing diabetes is usually between 37 and 38+6 weeks' gestation if no complications are present or before 37 weeks' gestation if there are complications.[1]

The aim of intrapartum care is to promote maternal and fetal well-being and optimize the childbirth experience for the woman, whilst ensuring safety.

Women with diabetes may need steroids for fetal lung maturation in preterm birth, and additional insulin to manage this may be given according to an agreed protocol.[1]

Women should be encouraged to express and store colostrum milk prior to delivery, known as breastmilk harvesting. Women need to discuss with their specialist team first, as this will be dependent on gestation.[2]

During labour and birth, women should have blood their glucose level measured every hour and maintained between 4 and 7mmol/L.[2] The Joint British Diabetes Societies (2023)[3] acknowledge that glucose levels of 5–8mmol/L may offer an acceptable margin of safety, but this currently has a limited evidence base.

Variable-rate insulin infusion (VRII) should be considered for women with T1D or T2D or those with GDM who are not maintaining glucose levels between 4 and 7mmol/L.[1] For guidance on appropriate variable-rate insulin infusions, refer to local or national guidelines.[3]

Continuation of CSII therapy during labour and birth appears efficacious and safe, and the suggestion is that this should be standard practice if the woman is able to self-manage this.[4]

References

1. National Institute for Health and Care Excellence (2015, updated 2020). *Diabetes in pregnancy: management from preconception to the postpartum period*. NICE guideline [NG3]. Available at: ℛ www.nice.org.uk/guidance/ng3
2. ABCD DTN-UK (2020). *Best practice guide: using diabetes technology in pregnancy*. Version 2.0. Available at: ℛ https://abcd.care/sites/default/files/site_uploads/Resources/DTN/BP-Pregnancy-DTN-V2.0.pdf
3. Joint British Diabetes Societies for Inpatient Care (2023). *Managing diabetes and hyperglycaemia during labour and birth*. Available at: ℛ https://abcd.care/sites/default/files/site_uploads/JBDS_Guidelines_Current/JBDS_12_Managing_diabetes_and_hyperglycaemia_during_labour_and_birth_with_QR_code_February_2023.pdf
4. Drever E, Tomlinson G, Bai AD, Feig DS. Insulin pump use compared with intravenous insulin during labour and delivery: the INSPIRED observational cohort study. *Diabetic Medicine*. 2016;**33**(9):1253–9.

Postnatal care

After delivery, women with diabetes may have additional needs when supporting them in adapting to parenthood. This will involve combining optimal glucose levels, whilst coping with the demands of a new baby. In women with pre-existing diabetes, insulin requirements drop immediately after birth and women are at ↑ risk of hypoglycaemia in the first few days after birth.[1]

Women with T1D will need a reduction in insulin doses immediately after birth, especially if breastfeeding. In women with other types of pre-existing diabetes, insulin may be stopped completely, although metformin may continue. In women with GDM, all glucose-lowering therapy is generally stopped.[2] The diabetes antenatal team will formulate a postnatal plan in partnership with the woman.

There is an ↑ risk of hypoglycaemia when breastfeeding, so it is important to ensure snacks are available when feeding or expressing breast milk. The aim is for glucose levels to be >6mmol/L.[1]

After delivery, babies should ideally be fed within 30 minutes of birth, then 2- to 3-hourly to prevent any neonatal hypoglycaemia.

If there is any neonatal hypoglycaemia with abnormal clinical signs, then the baby will need to be admitted to the neonatal specialist unit.

Babies should also receive specialist neonatal unit care if <34 weeks' gestation.

Babies should only be transferred to the care of community midwives when they are at least 24 hours old and satisfied that they are maintaining glucose levels and feeding.[2]

For all women with diabetes in pregnancy, ensure medications that were stopped before pregnancy are reviewed.[2]

Follow-up

Pre-existing diabetes

- For women with pre-existing diabetes, provide contact details for diabetes support and post-partum follow-up 6–12 weeks after delivery, then refer back to the usual diabetes team.
- For the first few weeks at least, there are challenges when caring for a new baby such as unpredictability, less routine, and less sleep. The emphasis should be on avoiding hypoglycaemia, and women may need support in transitioning to the recommended postnatal glucose targets of 3.9–10mmol/L.[1]
- Contraception and preconception advice for future pregnancies should also be discussed.

Gestational diabetes mellitus

- Check blood glucose levels postnatally and offer continued lifestyle advice, including offering referral to commissioned diabetes prevention programmes such as the NHS Diabetes Prevention Programme (see ➡ Chapter 2).
- Check a fasting glucose level 6–13 weeks postnatally or HbA1c after 13 weeks.
- Offer an annual HbA1c and ongoing diabetes prevention advice.

- Up to 50–60% of women with GDM may develop T2D in later life, so the above interventions provide an opportunity to intervene, aiming to prevent the development of T2D and provide for early optimal care in any future pregnancy.

References

1. ABCD DTN-UK (2020). *Best practice guide: using diabetes technology in pregnancy.* Version 2.0. Available at: ℜ https://abcd.care/sites/default/files/site_uploads/Resources/DTN/BP-Pregnancy-DTN-V2.0.pdf
2. National Institute for Health and Care Excellence (2015, updated 2020). *Diabetes in pregnancy: management from preconception to the postpartum period.* NICE guideline [NG3]. Available at: ℜ www.nice.org.uk/guidance/ng3

Non-diabetic hyperglycaemia

This refers to blood glucose levels that are above normal, but not in the diabetes range (i.e. HbA1c 42–47mmol/mol). At present, there is very little evidence to guide how this is managed in pregnancy and postnatally, but it has been highlighted that for these women, there is an ↑ risk of developing T2D in the future.[1]

Reference

1. Ravindrarajah R, Sutton M, Reeves D, *et al*. Referral to the NHS Diabetes Prevention Programme and conversion from nondiabetic hyperglycaemia to type 2 diabetes mellitus in England: a matched cohort analysis. *PLoS Medicine*. 2023;**20**(2):e1004177. Available at: ℘ https://doi.org/10.1371/journal.pmed.1004177

Perioperative management of diabetes

Introduction

Diabetes affects >15% of the surgical population. Surgical patients with diabetes have higher morbidity and mortality rates and longer hospital stays than patients without diabetes having the same procedure. There is clear evidence which suggests that the length of stay for people with diabetes is about 1 day longer than for those without diabetes.[1] One study found that a rise in plasma glucose level intraoperatively of 1mmol/L ↑ adverse events by 1.31-fold.[2] The physiological stress of surgery with the addition of anaesthetic agents can further raise plasma glucose levels and ↑ insulin resistance. If not treated appropriately, these may lead to diabetes emergencies such as diabetic ketoacidosis (DKA) or hyperosmolar hyperglycaemic state (HHS) (see ➜ Chapter 12). Perioperative hyperglycaemia is also associated with ↑ rates of infection (both surgical site infections and systemic infections such as urinary tract and lower respiratory tract infections) and medical complications, including acute kidney injury (AKI) (see ➜ Chapter 11), acute coronary syndromes, and acute cerebrovascular events. On the other hand, hypoglycaemia is associated with ↑ length of stay and inpatient mortality. The National Confidential Enquiry into Patient Outcome and Death (NCEPOD) published a report *Highs and Lows*, which highlighted several deficiencies within perioperative diabetes care around poor communication between specialties and lack of planning around diabetes management prior, during, and after surgery.[3]

References

1. Kerr M (2013). Inpatient care for people with diabetes: the economic case for change. Available at: ⌕ www.diabetes.nhs.uk/document.php?o=3034
2. Want J, Chen K, Li X, et al. Postoperative adverse events in patients with diabetes undergoing orthopedic and general surgery. *Medicine (Baltimore)*. 2019;**98**:e15089.
3. The National Confidential Enquiry into Patient Outcome and Death (2018). *Highs and lows*. Available at: ⌕ www.ncepod.org.uk/2018pd/Highs%20and%20Lows_Full%20Report.pdf

Elective surgery

Preoperative planning

Primary care referral

When referring for surgery/procedures, the referral letter should contain:

- Duration and type of diabetes
- Usual diabetes care team information
- Comorbidities
- Treatment
- Complications and their management
- Recent (within past 3 months) body mass index, blood pressure, HbA1c, and estimated glomerular filtration rate.

Aim for an *HbA1c of <69mmol/mol* before referral, if possible, and consider referral to the diabetes specialist team if diabetes optimization is safely achievable prior to surgery.[1]

Preoperative assessment

All patients undergoing an elective procedure must be referred to a pre-operative assessment clinic. Surgeons should ensure that patients with diabetes are not scheduled for an evening list to avoid unnecessary use of intravenous insulin infusions, prolonged fasting times, and an unnecessary overnight stay.

Preoperative assessment clinic staff should:

- Assess for adequacy of glycaemic levels
- Consider referral to the diabetes specialist team according to local policy
- Identify other comorbidities that require optimization before surgery
- Plan inpatient admission, including timing of surgery and pre-admission management of diabetes medications
- Consider the need for home support following discharge by liaising with primary care teams.

The risks of proceeding with surgery when glycaemic levels are suboptimal should be balanced against the urgency of the procedure.

For a suitable pathway for surgery based on HbA1c level, see Fig. 16.1.

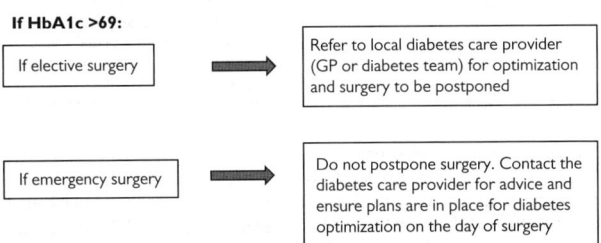

Fig. 16.1 Pathway to surgery based on HbA1c value.

Adjustment of diabetes medications
Patients should be given clear verbal and written instructions regarding which diabetes medications they should take the day before and on the day of surgery.

Insulins
Long-acting insulins should not be stopped during the perioperative period. Table 16.1 shows an example of preoperative adjustments for insulin (example of guidance by the Team at Manchester University Foundation Trust based on <u>Centre for Perioperative Care (2023)</u>. <u>*Guideline for perioperative care for people with diabetes mellitus undergoing elective and emergency surgery.*</u> <u>Available at:</u> ✆ www.cpoc.org.uk/sites/cpoc/files/documents/2024-03/CPOC-DiabetesGuideline2023.pdf).

Table 16.1 Example of preoperative adjustments for insulin (according to local hospital guideline)

Insulin	Day Prior to Surgery	Day of surgery
Long acting insulins (see ➋ chapter 5)	If normally taken in the morning, take usual dose If normally taken in the evening then take 80% of usual dose (0.8 x dose)	If normally taken in the morning, take 80% of usual dose If normally taken in the evening, give usual evening dose post-operatively
Biphasic or pre-mixed insulin (see ➋ chapter 5)	No dose change	Take 50% of usual morning dose Give usual evening dose post-operatively if eating a 'normal' meal. Give 50% of usual dose if eating a half/'small' meal
Short/rapid acting insulins (see ➋ chapter 5)	No dose change	**AM List** Omit morning short acting insulin dose Omit lunchtime short acting insulin if not eating. If eating a half/'small meal' then give 50% of usual dose **PM List** Take usual morning dose if having breakfast Omit lunchtime short acting insulin Give usual evening dose post-operatively if eating a 'normal' meal. Give 50% of usual dose if eating a half/'small' meal

Non-insulin diabetes medication
Table 16.2 shows an example of preoperative adjustments for non-insulin medications (example of guidance by the Team at Manchester University Foundation Trust based on <u>Centre for Perioperative Care (2023)</u>. <u>*Guideline for perioperative care for people with diabetes mellitus undergoing elective and emergency surgery.*</u> <u>Available at:</u> ✆ www.cpoc.org.uk/sites/cpoc/files/documents/2024-03/CPOC-DiabetesGuideline2023.pdf).

Table 16.2 Example of preoperative adjustments for non-insulin medications (according to local hospital guideline)

Medication	Day prior to surgery	Day of surgery for AM surgery	Day of surgery for PM surgery	While on a VRIII
Meglitinide	Take as normal	Omit morning dose	Give morning dose with breakfast	Stop until eating & drinking normally
Metformin (AND eGFR >60 ml/min/ 1.73m2 OR procedure not requiring use of contrast media)	Take as normal	If taken once or twice a day—take as normal If taken three times per day, omit lunchtime dose	If taken once or twice a day—take as normal If taken three times per day, omit lunchtime dose	Stop until eating & drinking normally and renal function stable (<25% fall in eGFR from baseline AND eGFR>30ml/ min/1.7m2)
Sulfonylurea	Take as normal	Once daily AM—omit Twice daily—omit morning dose and restart once eating and drinking normally	Once daily AM—omit Twice daily—omit morning dose and restart once eating and drinking normally	Stop until eating & drinking normally
Pioglitazone	Take as normal	Take as normal	Take as normal	Stop until eating & drinking normally
DPP IV Inhibitor (Gliptin)	Take as normal	Take as normal	Take as normal	Stop until eating & drinking normally

(Continued)

Table 16.2 (Contd.)

GLP-1 analogue/GLP1-GIP analogues (see paragraph below on perioperative use of GLP-1 RAs/ GLP1-GIP analogues and SGLT2-inhibitors)	Take as normal	Take as normal	Stop until eating & drinking normally
SGLT2 inhibitors (see paragraph below on perioperative use of GLP-1 RAs/ GLP1-GIP analogues and SGLT2-inhibitors)	Omit	Omit	Omit and only restart when the patient is clinically well and on full oral intake

Perioperative use of glucagon-like peptide-1 receptor agonists and glucose-dependent insulinotropic peptide and SGLT2 inhibitors

There are ongoing debates about the use of these medications in the perioperative period. The American Diabetes Association 'Standards of Care in Diabetes' guideline recommends stopping glucagon-like peptide 1 (GLP-1) receptor agonists the day prior to the procedure if taken daily and a week before if taken weekly, the reason being the ↑ risk of aspiration under anaesthesia.[2] But a recently published consensus statement recommends continuing these medications throughout the perioperative period.[3] The new recommendations include the need for a shared decision making approach with the patient to mitigate the risk of pulmonary aspiration.

In response to the risk of sodium–glucose cotransporter 2 (SGLT2) inhibitor-associated perioperative ketoacidosis, the US Food and Drug administration (FDA) recommendations are to stop these drugs at least 3–4 days before planned surgery.[4] But the new consensus statement published by British anesthetists recommends a shared decision making approach and the advice is to omit these drugs the day before and the day of a procedure.[3] It also recommends restarting these drugs once eating and drinking normally and with written sick day guidance provided during preoperative assessment and at discharge.

Intraoperative guidance

Frequency of capillary blood glucose monitoring

Check capillary blood glucose (CBG) on admission and then:
- Hourly if on insulin or insulin secretagogues such as sulfonylureas or meglitinides
- Two-hourly CBG for patients with diabetes NOT on insulin or insulin secretagogues.

Variable-rate intravenous insulin infusion

The main aim of a variable-rate intravenous insulin infusion (VRIII) is to maintain blood glucose levels within the target range of 6–10mmol/L, although up to 12mmol/L is also acceptable. A VRIII is set up by infusing a constant rate of glucose-containing fluid as substrate, while infusing insulin at a variable rate. Fig. 16.2 shows an example of a VRIII.[5]

Criteria for commencing VRIII include:
- Patients with type 1 diabetes (T1D) (including those on a continuous subcutaneous insulin infusion (CSII) (insulin pump) who will miss >1 meal
- Patients with T1D who have not received their long-acting insulin
- Patients with type 2 diabetes (T2D) who will miss >1 meal with CBG level of >12mmol/L
- Most patients having emergency surgery.

Consider VRIII for patients with HbA1c ≥69mmol/mol.
All surgical patients going to critical care will have VRIII commenced if blood glucose levels are above 10mmol/L.

Glucose (mmol/l)	Insulin rates (ml/h) Start on standard scale unless otherwise indicated				
	Reduced Rate Scale For use in insulin sensitive people with diabetes (frail older, renal patients or those who usually need less than 24 units per day)	Standard Scale (First choice in most cases)	**Increased Rate Scale** For use in insulin resistant people with diabetes— (Patients using > 100 units per day preadmission or with BMI > 35 kg/m^2)	Custo- mised Scale	Custo- mised Scale
NB If patient is on basal insulin, continue basal insulin.					
< 6.0	0*	0*	0*		
6.1 to 8.0	0.5	1	2		
8.1 to 11.0	1	2	4		
11.1 to 15.0	2	4	6		
15.1 to 20.0	3	5	7		
20.1 to 28.0	4	6	8		
28.1 or more	6	8	10		

Fig. 16.2 Example of a variable-rate intravenous insulin infusion.

General guidance
- Blood glucose level must be checked prior to induction of anaesthesia and should be recorded on the anaesthetic record.
- Handover from recovery to the ward nurse should include any diabetes medications given in theatre, blood glucose level on leaving the recovery area, and prescription for diabetes medications.

Post-operative guidance

Patients should resume self-management of their diabetes where appropriate and as soon as possible after surgery.

- For patients not on VRIII, diabetes medication should be restarted with their next meal at the preoperative doses and regime, unless the patient is not able to eat and drink normally (see Tables 16.1 and 16.2 for guidance).
- For patients with T1D on VRIII, transition from intravenous to subcutaneous insulin should take place when the next meal-related dose is due. Insulin should be given with a meal, and the VRIII can be stopped 30 minutes later. If the long-acting insulin was stopped perioperatively in error, the VRIII should be continued until a dose of this is given.
- For patients on CSII, they can restart their pump once they are able to manage it by themselves. There needs to be an overlap of 60 minutes from recommencing their CSII pump and stopping the VRIII.
- For patients with T2D on VRIII, diabetes medications should be restarted with their next meal unless the patient is not able to eat and drink. Dose reductions may be needed if the patient is taking small amount of food and fluids.

Once VRIII is discontinued, monitor CBG levels hourly for at least 2 hours and if in acceptable range, revert to local glucose monitoring policy.

Be aware that diabetes medication doses may need adjusting because of post-operative stress, infection, and altered food intake.

Consult the inpatient diabetes team if recurrent hyper- or hypoglycaemia.

References

1. JBDS (2019). Joint British Diabetes Societies for Inpatient Care. A good inpatient diabetes service. Available at: ℘ https://abcd.care/sites/default/files/site_uploads/JBDS_Guidelines_Current/JBDS_14_A_Good_Inpatient_Service_Updated_060720.pdf. Accessed March 2024.
2. American Diabetes Association Professional Practice Committee (2024). 16. Diabetes care in the hospital: standards of care in diabetes. Available at: ℘ https://diabetesjournals.org/care/article/47/Supplement_1/S295/153950/16-Diabetes-Care-in-the-Hospital-Standards-of-Care
3. Anaesthesia (2025). Elective peri-operative management of adults taking glucagon-like peptide-1 receptor agonists, glucose-dependent insulinotropic peptide agonists and sodium-glucose cotransporter-2 inhibitors: a multidisciplinary consensus statement. Available at: ℘ https://associationofanaesthetists-publications.onlinelibrary.wiley.com/doi/epdf/10.1111/anae.16541
4. US Food and Drug Administration (2022). FDA revises labels of SGLT2 inhibitors for diabetes to include warnings about too much acid in the blood and serious urinary tract infections. Available at: ℘ www.fda.gov/Drugs/DrugSafety/ucm475463.htm
5. Centre for Perioperative Care (2023). Guideline for perioperative care for people with diabetes mellitus undergoing elective and emergency surgery. Available at: ℘ www.cpoc.org.uk/sites/cpoc/files/documents/2024-03/CPOC-DiabetesGuideline2023.pdf

Emergency surgery

All patients with diabetes having an emergency surgical admission should have their blood glucose levels and metabolic status documented on admission.

- For patients with T1D, ketone levels must be checked and insulin prescribed. Assess for the need for VRIII, especially for people with poor glycaemic control and patients on CSII.
- For patients with T2D, ensure SGLT2 inhibitors are withheld and ketone levels are checked. Assess for the need for VRIII, especially if blood glucose levels are above 12mmol/L.

Post-operatively, diabetes medications should be started, according to the guidance shown in Tables 16.1 and 16.2.

The Getting it Right for the First Time (GIRFT) team has developed a diabetes emergency surgery pathway[1] (see Fig. 16.3).

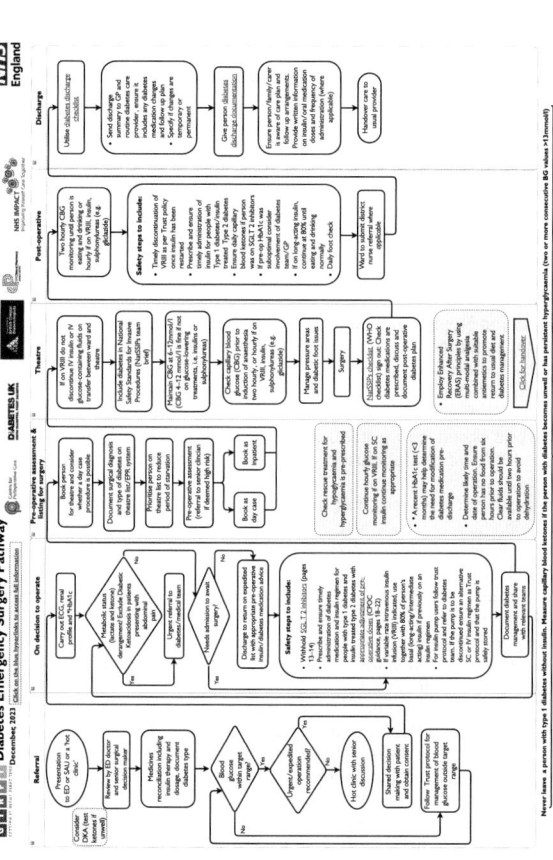

Fig. 16.3 With kind permission to use by the GIRFT Team.

Pathway for diabetes emergency surgery available at ℗ https://getingrightfirsttime.co.uk/wp-content/uploads/2023/12/Diabetes-Emergency-Surgery-Pathway-FINAL-V1-December-2023.html

Management of patients on continuous subcutaneous insulin infusion pumps

Prior to admission

- Patients should contact their local insulin pump team for review prior to surgery.
- All patients on a hybrid closed loop insulin pump system need to check with their diabetes team if it is appropriate to use this system for surgery[2].
- Patients should replace their pump cannula on the day before surgery.
- The reservoir should be full of insulin, and new or recently replaced batteries should be in place.
- The cannula should have been sited well away from the area of the surgery (at least 15cm if possible) and in a site still accessible by the theatre team (not on the back or buttocks, unless it has been instructed to do so by the diabetes care provider or surgical team).
- Patients should continue their pump at the usual basal rate and self-correct to blood glucose levels of 6–10mmol/L.[2,3]

On admission

- Hourly blood glucose checks from admission.
- Check the pump site for disconnection/kinking preoperatively, perioperatively, and in recovery.
- Blood glucose checks at least hourly while sedated/under general anaesthesia.
- If on hybrid closed loop system, advise the patient to switch to activity/exercise/ease-off mode prior to surgery to prevent hypoglycaemia during sedation.[1]
- The anaesthetist/recovery staff should NOT give boluses via the CSII pump.
- If glucose levels are >12mmol/L or if the patient will miss >1 meal, start VRIII and remove the pump.
- If hypoglycaemia, treat initially as per local guidance. If persistent hypoglycaemia occurs, continue to treat as per local guidance and remove the pump cannula and pump. Once normoglycaemic, restart insulin, either with CSII if the patient is now alert and able to self-manage or with VRIII.
- If the CSII pump alarm sets off during the procedure, do not attempt to rectify; monitor CBG levels every 30 minutes and start VRIII if >12mmol/L. If the CSII alarm becomes intrusive, remove the CSII pump and cannula and store safely.
- To minimize the risk of electromagnetic interference with diathermy and the CSII pump, use bipolar diathermy, where possible, and the lowest effective diathermy settings for electrocautery.[2,3]

Post-operatively

- Continue with hourly CBGs until eating and drinking.
- Once alert and orientated post-operatively, the patient should self-correct to a CBG level of 6–10mmol/L if in open loop.

- If using a hybrid closed loop system, switch to activity/exercise/ease-off mode[2]
- The patient can then recommence mealtime boluses once eating and drinking normally.[2,3]

References

1. Diabetes Emergency Surgery Pathway (2023). ℅ https://gettingitrightfirsttime.co.uk/wp-content/uploads/2023/12/Diabetes-Emergency-Surgery-Pathway-FINAL-V1-December-2023.html
2. Partridge H, Perkins B, Mathieu S, Nicholls A, Adeniji K. Clinical recommendations in the management of the patient with type 1 diabetes on insulin pump therapy in the perioperative period: a primer for the anaesthetist. *British Journal of Anaesthesia*. 2016;**116**(1):18–26.
3. Diabetes Technology Network (2018). *Guidelines for managing continuous subcutaneous insulin infusion (CSII, or 'insulin pump') therapy in hospitalised patients*. Available at: ℅ https://abcd.care/sites/default/files/CSII_DTN_FINAL%20210218.pdf

Management of hyperglycaemia

The main causes for perioperative hyperglycaemia include:
- Hospital-acquired DKA or HHS
- Stress hyperglycaemia
- Insufficient delivery of diabetes medications
- Sepsis.

For patients who are not managed on VRIII:[1]
- Check that all diabetes medications are prescribed and given.
- Treat any nausea and vomiting.
- Assess for DKA by checking for ketones and venous blood gas levels.
- If on CSII, patients should be encouraged to take bolus doses of insulin to correct hyperglycaemia. If two doses of bolus insulin do not work, consider commencing VRIII and stop the CSII pump.
- If not in DKA, correct hyperglycaemia with subcutaneous rapid-acting insulin; 1 unit of rapid-acting insulin to reduce the CBG level by ~3mmol/L. Aim for CBG levels of around 8mmol/L. Give a maximum of 6 units subcutaneously by using a specific insulin syringe.
- Check CBG levels hourly. Consider a second dose of insulin after 2 hours.
- If two doses of subcutaneous insulin do not work, consider commencing VRIII.
- Contact the inpatient diabetes team for advice.

Reference

1. Diabetes-Perioperative Guideline (2021). Perioperative Diabetes Guidelines—Management of adult patients with diabetes having surgery (or any procedure requiring a period of fasting. Available at: ℛ https://intranet.mft.nhs.uk/documents/policies/1659

Management of hypoglycaemia

Where a hypoglycaemic episode is >2 hours from the estimated surgical start time, use a clear sugar-containing drink, for example:
- 200mL of apple juice or pulp-free orange juice OR
- 4–5 glucose tablets or 5–6 dextrose tablets or glucose gel.

Where a hypoglycaemic episode is <2 hours from the estimated surgical start time, avoid the oral route. Use intravenous dextrose or intramuscular glucagon:
- 150mL of 10% glucose intravenously OR 1mg of glucagon intramuscularly (where intravenous access is difficult)
- Recheck the blood glucose level 15 minutes after treatment, and repeat the steps if necessary.[1]

Looming hypoglycaemia

This is defined as a CBG level of between 4 and 6mmol/L in a person with diabetes who is on a glucose-lowering medication such as sulfonylureas and meglitinides. Consider initiating hypoglycaemia treatment, particularly if the patient is sedated or anaesthetized.

Do not treat CBG levels of 4–6mmol/L if the patient is diet-controlled or on oral antidiabetic medications which do not cause hypoglycaemia (e.g. metformin or dipeptidyl dipeptidase type 4 (DPP-4) inhibitors).

When to check for blood ketones

- If a patient with diabetes becomes unwell.
- If a patient has persistent hyperglycaemia (two or more consecutive CBG values >13mmol/L).
- Daily if the patient is normally on SGLT2 inhibitors (gliflozins), even if glucose levels are normal.
- Emergency surgical patients on admission.
- In a patient with T1D prior to discontinuing VRIII (ensure blood ketone levels are <0.6mmol/L prior to discontinuing VRIII).

Reference

1. Diabetes-Perioperative Guideline (2021). Perioperative Diabetes Guidelines—Management of adult patients with diabetes having surgery (or any procedure requiring a period of fasting. Available at: ℛ https://intranet.mft.nhs.uk/documents/policies/1659

Getting It Right First Time

Getting It Right First Time (GIRFT) is a national programme that was initiated in 2016 and designed to improve medical care within the National Health Service (NHS) by reducing unwarranted variations.[1] The programme identified changes that can help to improve care and patient outcomes, as well as deliver efficiencies such as reduction of unnecessary procedures and cost savings. GIRFT encourages trusts and local systems to consider and tailor best practice pathways to their population needs.

The GIRFT diabetes work stream is focused on helping people with diabetes and their clinicians in effectively managing the condition and reducing avoidable harms.

Improving the Perioperative Pathway for Patients with Diabetes (IP3D)

GIRFT data showed considerable variation in length of stay for patients with diabetes undergoing surgery. In some hospitals, this excess length of stay was seen to be as many as 4.5 days. Even though there were several guidelines that existed around the management of perioperative diabetes, their implementation was found particularly challenging. GIRFT identified several opportunities to ↑ patient experience and staff education within the area of perioperative diabetes management.

In 2019, a project was implemented at Ipswich Hospital, part of East Suffolk and North Essex NHS Foundation Trust—*Improving the Perioperative Pathway for Patients with Diabetes* (the IP3D project), which yielded positive outcomes for patients with diabetes undergoing surgery and considerable reduction in length of hospital stay.[2]

The key recommendations of this project are:

- Introduction of a perioperative patient passport that is designed to empower the patient along their surgical journey by providing them with all the necessary information required before, during, and after their surgery and can be used as a resource between patient and clinicians involved in their care (see Fig. 16.4 for an example of a patient passport).
- Appointment of a perioperative diabetes specialist nurse (Perioperative DSN) who provides education and support to patients both pre- and post-operatively, as well as working with surgical staff to improve diabetes education.
- The Perioperative DSN to attend weekly huddles in various preoperative assessment units and to work on improving several processes in the perioperative pathway.
- The introduction of preoperative diabetes optimization clinics to improve glycaemic levels of patients with HbA1c >69mmol/mol, awaiting elective surgery.
- Facilitation of annual surgical study days, with each surgical area having its own dedicated surgical diabetes link nurse/champions who links in regularly with the perioperative diabetes nurse.
- Development of a robust audit protocol to measure clinical outcomes.

The pathway showed considerable improvement in perioperative outcomes for people with diabetes undergoing surgery, with the potential for cost savings.

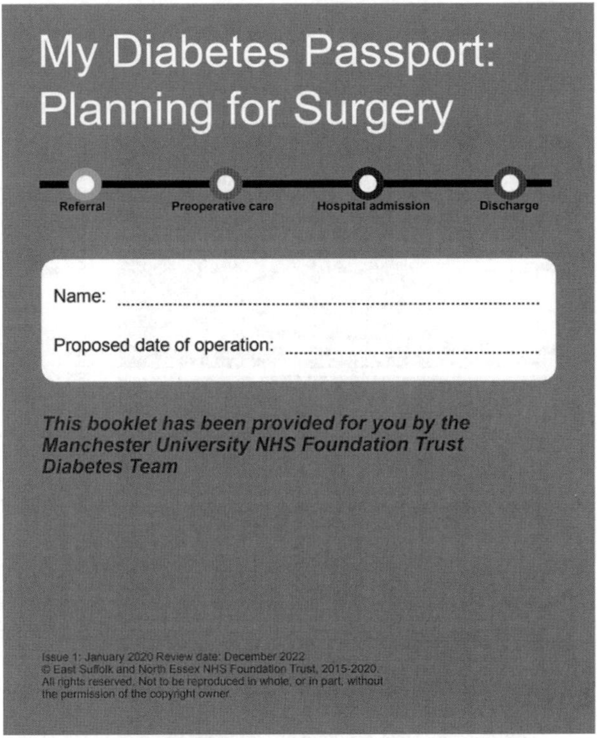

Fig. 16.4 Example of a patient passport.

This booklet has been produced by the team at Manchester University Foundation Trust based on the resource of the IP3Dteam.

The IP3D project was independently evaluated and was found to have led to:
- A 71% reduction in patients with diabetes who experienced diabetes-related harm or complications such as hyper- and hypoglycaemic events, foot ulcers, DKA, and poor wound healing
- Reduced length of stay by 1.5 days for elective surgery inpatients with diabetes
- A better experience for patients, according to post-surgery survey
- Improved staff knowledge, particularly around hyperglycaemia management.

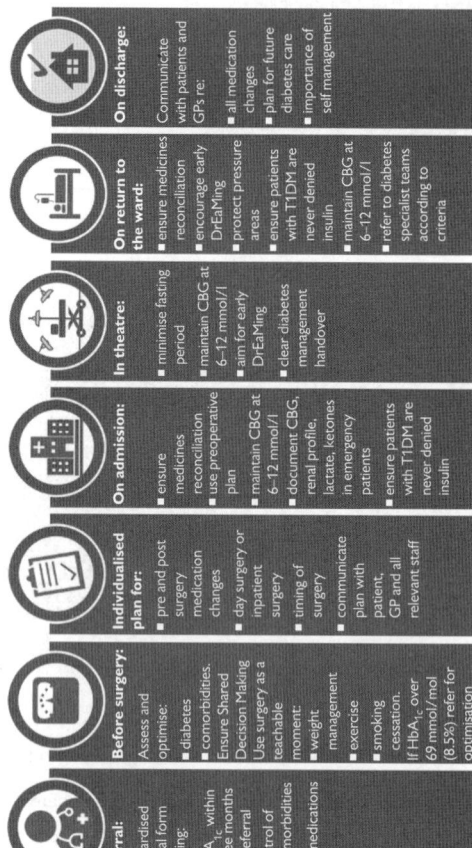

Referral:

Standardised referral form including:
- HbA1c within three months of referral
- control of co-morbidities
- all medications

Before surgery:

Assess and optimise:
- diabetes
- comorbidities.

Ensure Shared Decision Making

Use surgery as a teachable moment:
- weight management
- exercise
- smoking cessation.

If HbA1c over 69 mmol/mol (8.5%) refer for optimisation

Individualised plan for:
- pre and post surgery medication changes
- day surgery or inpatient surgery
- timing of surgery
- communicate plan with patient, GP and all relevant staff

On admission:
- ensure medicines reconciliation
- use preoperative plan
- maintain CBG at 6-12 mmol/l
- document CBG, renal profile, lactate, ketones in emergency patients
- ensure patients with T1DM are never denied insulin

In theatre:
- minimise fasting period
- maintain CBG at 6-12 mmol/l
- aim for early DrEaMing
- clear diabetes management handover

On return to the ward:
- ensure medicines reconciliation
- encourage early DrEaMing
- protect pressure areas
- ensure patients with T1DM are never denied insulin
- maintain CBG at 6-12 mmol/l
- refer to diabetes specialist teams according to criteria

On discharge:

Communicate with patients and GPs re:
- all medication changes
- plan for future diabetes care
- importance of self management

CBG = capillary blood glucose

Shared Decision Making = the process whereby patients and clinicians work together to make evidenced based decisions centred on patient values and preferences-including risks, benefits, alternatives and optimisation.

T1DM = Type 1 Diabetes Mellitus

DrEaMing = Drinking, Eating and Mobilising

Fig. 16.5 The perioperative pathway for people with diabetes undergoing elective and emergency surgery.

The project has since been rolled out to further trusts across England and has shown improved outcomes and experience for people with diabetes undergoing surgery.

References

1. NHS England. *Getting It Right First Time (GIRFT)*. Available at: ℗ https://gettingitrightfirsttime.co.uk
2. NHS England. *Improving the Perioperative Pathway for Patients with Diabetes*. Available at: ℗ https://gettingitrightfirsttime.co.uk/associated_projects/improving-the-perioperative-pathway-for-patients-with-diabetes

Further reading

Dhatariya K, Brown P (2022). *How to prepare people with diabetes for surgery*. Available at: ℗ https://diabetesonthenet.com/diabetes-primary-care/how-to-prepare-people-with-diabetes-for-surgery-2022
Dhatariya K, Levy N, Russon K, *et al*. Perioperative use of glucagon-like peptide-1 receptor agonists and sodium-glucose cotransporter 2 inhibitors for diabetes mellitus. *British Journal of Anaesthesia*. 2024;**132**(4):639–43. Available at: ℗ www.sciencedirect.com/science/article/pii/S0007091223007316?via%3Dihub

Case study

Mrs Akhtar is a 60-year-old lady with type 2 diabetes, listed for coronary artery bypass graft surgery as an elective procedure. During the preoperative assessment, her HbA1c has been reported as 85mmol/mol. Her current diabetes medications include metformin 1g twice daily, gliclazide 160mg twice daily, alogliptin 25mg once daily, and empagliflozin 25mg once daily. Her current diabetes care provider is the general practitioner (GP).

The cardiac surgical team has cancelled the surgery in view of raised HbA1c.

Question 1

What measures can be implemented to ensure Mrs Akhtar has safe surgery, with no post-operative complications?

Answers

- Speak to Mrs Akhtar to make sure she is taking her prescribed diabetes medications regularly.
- Optimization of HbA1c prior to surgery. Check if the hospital diabetes team has a preoperative diabetes optimization clinic and refer Mrs Akhtar to this service. If this service is not available, request the GP to optimize her glucose levels by initiating insulin therapy or by completing an urgent referral to the local diabetes care team provider for the same.
- Recheck HbA1c 3 months after initiation of insulin therapy.
- Inform the surgical team once HbA1c is below 69mmol/mol.

Mrs Akhtar was referred to the preoperative diabetes optimization clinic and was started on regular insulin therapy. Her current diabetes medications include metformin 1g twice daily, Humulin I® insulin 38 units in the morning and 24 units in the evening, and empagliflozin 25mg once daily. HbA1c was rechecked after 3 months and has been reported now as 64mmol/mol. The surgical team has relisted her for surgery and she is on an early morning surgical list. Nil by mouth from 12 midnight.

Question 2

What advice must be given to Mrs Akhtar in preparation for surgery?

Answers

- Diabetes medication dose changes:
  - Metformin to be omitted the day before and on the day of surgery
  - Empagliflozin to be omitted the day before and on the day of surgery
  - 80% dose of Humulin I® to be taken the day before and on the morning of surgery.
- Blood glucose levels to be checked hourly from 6 a.m. on the day of surgery. Treat hypoglycaemia with oral agents up to 2 hours prior to surgery.

Question 3

How to ensure Mrs Akhtar's diabetes is managed effectively whilst in hospital?

Answers

- Hourly CBG checks from the time of admission.
- Treat hypoglycaemia as per trust policy.
- If CBG levels are above 12mmol/L, commence VRIII.
- Restart regular diabetes medications once eating and drinking well. Check blood ketone levels before restarting empagliflozin.
- If on VRIII post-surgery, commence regular diabetes medications and stop VRIII 30 minutes after this.
- Contact the inpatient diabetes team for advice and support, if needed.
- Ensure safe discharge planning. The discharge summary should include information about current diabetes medications, any dose changes, and request for continued diabetes team support in the community.

Other important areas of diabetes care

Ramadan

Ramadan fasting (or sawm) is one of the Five Pillars of Islam, considered by believers to be the foundation of Muslim life.

Fasting occurs in the ninth month of the Islamic calendar (Hijra).

The Islamic calendar is lunar-based and has only 354 days. It therefore occurs 11 days earlier each year.

Ramadan has great religious and cultural importance for Muslims. Therefore, health care professionals (HCPs) need to understand the impact this has on people with diabetes.

Worldwide, ~116 million people with diabetes fast during Ramadan.[1]
- Fasting entails abstinence from food, liquid, and oral medications.
- The fasting period occurs between sunrise (suhoor) and sunset (iftar).
- Ramadan lasts for 29–30 days.
- In the UK, a fast lasts for 10–21 hours, depending on the season in which Ramadan falls.

All healthy individuals after puberty should fast.

Those for whom fasting is detrimental to their health are exempt from doing so. These include:
- Frail and elderly people
- Children
- Pregnant and breastfeeding women
- People with other long-term conditions.

Fig. 17.1 shows the British Islamic Medical Association's risk categories and recommendations for people with diabetes who fast during Ramadan.[2]

During Ramadan, a person with diabetes who decides to fast can be at risk of:
- Hypoglycaemia
- Hyperglycaemia
- Dehydration and thrombosis
- Diabetic ketoacidosis (DKA), including euglycaemic DKA
- Hyperosmolar hyperglycaemic state (HHS).

The landmark study Epidemiology of Diabetes and Ramadan (EPIDIAR)[4] found that during Ramadan, there was a 4.7- and 7.5-fold ↑ in the incidence of severe hypoglycaemic complications in people with type 1 diabetes (T1D) and type 2 diabetes (T2D), respectively, compared with non-Ramadan periods.

Ramadan-related diabetes education

Should ideally take place 1–2 months before fasting period starts and include:
- *Blood glucose monitoring*: it is advisable to check blood glucose levels several times a day if taking insulin and/or a sulfonylurea, as suggested below (this does not constitute breaking the fast):
  - Pre-dawn meal (suhoor)
  - Morning
  - Midday
  - Mid afternoon
  - Pre-sunset meal (iftar)

British Islamic Medical Association's* risk categories and recommendations for people with diabetes who fast during Ramadan.		
Risk category and religious opinion on fasting (boxed)*	Person characteristics	Comments
Category 1: **very high risk** **Religious opinion:** Listen to medical advice. MUST NOT fast.	One or more of the following: • Poorly controlled type 1 diabetes • Acute hyperglycaemic diabetes complications within the 3 months prior to Ramadan (DKA, HHS) • Disabling hypoglycaemia: severe hypoglycaemia within the 3 months prior to Ramadan, history of hypoglycaemia unawareness, recurrent hypoglycaemia • T2D requiring insulin (MDI or biphasic insulin therapy) with **no** prior experience of safe fasting • Advanced macrovascular complications • Chronic dialysis or CKD stages 4 and 5 • Pregnancy in pre-existing diabetes, or GDM† treated with insulin or SUs • Acute illness • Old age with ill health	If individual insists on fasting, then they should: • Receive structured education • Be followed by a qualified diabetes team and have access for advice during fasting • Check their blood glucose regularly (SMBG) • Adjust medication dose as per recommendations • Be prepared to break the fast in case of hypo- or hyperglycaemia
Category 2: **high risk** **Religious opinion:** Listen to medical advice. SHOULD NOT fast.	One or more of the following: • Well-controlled T1D • T2D with sustained poor glycaemic control** • T2D requiring insulin (MDI or biphasic insulin therapy) with prior experience of safe fasting • T2D on SGLT2 inhibitors (consider alternatives/pausing during Ramadan) • Stable macrovascular complications of diabetes • CKD stage 3 • Women with T2D who are pregnant or GDM controlled by diet only or metformin • People with comorbid conditions that present additional risk factors • Treatment with drugs that may affect cognitive function • People with diabetes performing intense physical labour	• Be prepared to stop the fast in case of frequent hypo- or hyperglycaemia or worsening of other related medical conditions
Category 3: **moderate/low risk** **Religious opinion:** Listen to medical advice. Decision to use licence not to fast based on discretion of medical opinion and ability of the individual to tolerate fast.	Well-controlled T2D treated with one or more of the following: • Diet and lifestyle therapy • Metformin • Incretin-based therapies (DPP-4 inhibitors, GLP-1 receptor agonists) • Thiazolidinedione (pioglitazone) • Acarbose • Second-generation SUs (moderate risk: regular SMBG advised) • Basal insulin (moderate risk: regular SMBG advised)	People who fast should: • Receive structured education • Check their blood glucose regularly (SMBG) • Adjust medication dose as per recommendations

*In each category, people with diabetes should follow medical opinion if the advice is not to fast due to high probability of harm.
**Consider HbA$_{1c}$ >75 mmol/mol for over 12 months.
If there is uncertainty about which group an individual falls into and they seek to fast, chapter 5 of the IDF/DAR guidelines† includes a risk calculator.
CKD=chronic kidney disease; DKA=diabetic ketoacidosis; GDM=gestational diabetes mellitus; HSS=hypersomolar hyperglycaemic state; SGLT2=sodium-glucose cotransporter 2; SMBG=self-monitoring of blood glucose; SUs=sulfonylureas; T1D=type 1 diabetes; T2D=type 2 diabetes.

Fig. 17.1 British Islamic Medical Association's risk categories and recommendations for people with diabetes who fast during Ramadan.[3]
Taken from Gilani A (2023) How to manage diabetes in Ramadan. *Diabetes & Primary Care* **25**: 27–92.

- 2 hours after iftar
- Any time when symptoms of hypo- or hyperglycaemia or feeling unwell.

(NB ensure access to continuous glucose monitoring (CGM) for those eligible)

- When to break fast:
  - If blood glucose levels are <3.9 or >16.7mmol/L
  - If there are symptoms of hypoglycaemia
  - An acute illness occurs.
- Exercise:
  - Light-to-moderate exercise.
- Dietary advice:[1]

Table 17.1 Recommended medication adjustments during Ramadan

Metformin	*Daily dose remains unchanged* *Immediate release:* • Daily—take at iftar • Twice daily—take at iftar and suhoor *Prolonged release:* • Take at iftar
SGLT2 inhibitors	No dose modifications Dose should be taken with iftar Extra clear fluids should be taken during non-fasting periods Use with caution in those at risk of fluid depletion
Sulfonylurea	Once daily—take at iftar. Dose should be reduced/stopped in people with lower glycaemic levels Twice daily—iftar dose remains unchanged. Suhoor dose should be reduced in people with lower glycaemic levels
Thiazolidinediones	No dose modifications Dose can be taken with iftar or suhoor
GLP-1RAs	No dose modifications
DPP-4 inhibitors	No dose modifications
Insulin	High risk of hypoglycaemia *Basal (long-acting) insulin:* • Preferred initial formulation • Dose reduction by 20% • Take at iftar *Rapid-acting insulin:* • Omit lunch dose • Take twice daily with meals at suhoor and iftar *Mixed insulin:* • Consider reducing doses, based on blood glucose readings and dietary patterns at iftar and suhoor

SGLT2, sodium–glucose cotransporter 2; GLP-1, glucagon-like peptide 1; DPP-4, dipeptidyl dipeptidase type 4.

For further information on insulin dose adjustments in Ramadan, see also *Diabetes and Ramadan: Practical Guidelines 2021*.[1]

- Encourage low-glycaemic index (GI), high-fibre foods for slow energy release.
- Begin iftar with 1–2 dates to raise blood glucose levels, and plenty of water to overcome dehydration.
- Avoid other sugary foods.
- Eat balanced meals: 45–50% carbohydrate, 20–30% protein, and <35% fat.
- Take suhoor as late as possible.
- Maintain hydration with water and non-sweetened beverages overnight between iftar and suhoor.
- Eat foods that induce satiety (i.e. with protein and fibre).
- Medication adjustment (see Table 17.1):[5]
  - During Ramadan, choose antidiabetes agents that have a lower risk of hypoglycaemia where possible.
  - New medications should ideally be initiated 6–8 weeks prior to Ramadan.

References

1. International Diabetes Federation (IDF), Diabetes and Ramadan (DAR) International Alliance (2021). *Diabetes and Ramadan: Practical Guidelines 2021.* Available at: ℜ https://pubmed.ncbi.nlm.nih.gov/35016991/
2. British Islamic Medical Association (2020). *Ramadan rapid review and recommendations: risk table and recommendations summary.* Available at: ℜ https://britishima.org/advice/ramadan-rapid-review
3. Gilani A. How to manage diabetes in Ramadan. *Diabetes & Primary Care.* 2023;**25**:27–9. Available at: ℜ https://diabetesonthenet.com/diabetes-primary-care/how-to-manage-diabetes-during-ramadan-march-2023
4. Salti I, Bénard E, Detournay B, *et al.*; EPIDIAR study group. A population-based study of diabetes and its characteristics during the fasting month of Ramadan in 13 countries: results of the epidemiology of diabetes and Ramadan 1422/2001 (EPIDIAR) study. *Diabetes Care.* 2004;**27**(10):2306–11.
5. Ibrahim M, Davies MJ, Ahmad E, *et al.* Recommendations for management of diabetes during Ramadan: update 2020, applying the principles of the ADA/EASD consensus. *BMJ Open Diabetes Research and Care.* 2020;**8**:e001248.

Travel and diabetes

All travel should ideally begin with planning and preparation.

Normal travel health advice is still applicable, and all recommendations regarding immunizations and antimalarials should be followed. This should include an assessment of any contraindications for antimalarials based on existing/past medical conditions or current medication.

Useful advice

Check with the airline or other operator for their guidelines for people living with diabetes.

Carry information, including:

- A list of all prescribed medications
- A list of necessary monitoring equipment and technology
- Letter by a HCP advising on the necessity of carrying medication, insulin, needles, syringes, sensors, and so forth, in hand luggage
- Download a Medical Device Awareness Card from the Civil Aviation Authority website if using any diabetes technology
- Contact details of the diabetes team in case information or advice is needed whilst away
- Travel insurance details
- Diabetes medical alert bracelet/insulin passport.

Packing

- Take enough medication to cover unexpected delays, damages, or losses (carried in hand luggage).
- Take spare monitoring equipment with supplies and batteries (carried in hand luggage), including, where appropriate, extra infusion sets and cannulae (for insulin pumps).
- All medications should be kept in their original packaging and carried in hand luggage to avoid loss or damage in the hold of the aircraft.
  - Insulin must be carried in hand luggage to avoid becoming too cold (and potentially freezing) in the hold.
  - Medications (including insulin) may be available under different trade names in other countries. Advise on the generic name of medications, in addition to their brand name.
- Carrying extra food and snacks, including fast-acting carbohydrates (hypoglycaemia treatment where applicable) to ensure adequate intake or to supplement airline food—this is particularly important if delayed flights are experienced.
- If travelling long haul through time zones and on insulin, it is recommended to discuss any changes to insulin doses and timing with the HCP well in advance of the planned travel date.

Technology

- If using technology (e.g. CGM or insulin pumps), consult the manufacturer's advice on flying with that device, especially as not all diabetes technology can safely go through airport security scanners.
- Insulin pumps and CGM are safe for use during air travel by using Bluetooth. They will still work when a phone is in flight mode.

During travel
- Monitor blood glucose levels more frequently due to the change in mealtimes and activity levels, especially on long-haul flights.
- Keep watch and devices set to country of origin times until landing.
- If taking insulin and travelling through multiple time zones for longer than 4 hours:
  - Travelling east to west will generally require more insulin.
  - Travelling west to east will generally require less insulin.
- When travelling with insulin, it is best to keep it cool by storing it in a fridge at destination or in a cool bag during travel (providing it does not freeze). A variety of cool bags and storage containers are available.

Effects of temperature

Hot climate
- Prolonged sun exposure may raise blood glucose levels; however, heat can also ↑ the risk of hypoglycaemia.
- Dehydration is a risk in very hot weather and is heightened if blood glucose levels are also high.
- Peripheral neuropathy: watch for unawareness of sunburn and hot surfaces; always wear shoes on hot sand or around the poolside.
- Raised temperatures can affect insulin storage, absorption, and glucose monitoring.

Cold climate
- Low blood glucose levels are more common in cold weather, as the body uses more energy to maintain its temperature.
- Low blood glucose levels are more dangerous in cold climates due to the risk of hypothermia.
- Peripheral neuropathy: watch for frostbite.
- Lower temperatures can affect insulin storage, absorption. and glucose monitoring.

NB persons travelling to areas of high altitude need careful and specialist planning, including relating to ↑ risk of hypoglycaemia and mountain sickness, and precautions for their prevention and effective management.

Diabetes complications, such as retinopathy, nephropathy, and neuropathy, should be assessed before travelling as each may be worsened by, or affect the body's acclimatization to, altitude.

Further reading

National Travel Health Network and Centre (NaTHNaC). *TravelHealthPro*. For travel health advice. Available at: ℘ https://travelhealthpro.org.uk

Public Health Scotland. *Fit For Travel*. Information on how to stay safe and healthy abroad. Available at: ℘ www.fitfortravel.nhs.uk/home

Trend Diabetes. *Diabetes and travel*. Available at: ℘ https://trenddiabetes.online/portfolio/diabetes-and-travel

Driving and diabetes

Provided a person meets the requirements for driving and does not have other complications which would affect their ability to drive (e.g. visual impairment, cardiac/renal conditions, or neuropathic exclusions), the following Driver and Vehicle Licensing Agency (DVLA) regulations apply (see Table 17.2).[1]

Driving and insulin

By law, the DVLA must be informed if any of the following applies:
- The individual experiences >1 episode of severe hypoglycaemia within the last 12 months while awake.
  - (For group 1 drivers, episodes of hypoglycaemia occurring during established sleep are no longer considered relevant for licensing

Table 17.2 DVLA (2024) Guidance for driving and diabetes medications

Treatment	Group 1 driver	Group 2 driver
Diabetes managed by diet/lifestyle alone	May drive and need not notify DVLA	May drive and need not notify DVLA
Managed by medication not associated with causing hypoglycaemia (metformin, DPP-4 inhibitors, pioglitazone, SGLT2 inhibitors, GLP-1RAs)	May drive and need not notify DVLA	May drive but <u>must</u> notify DVLA No need for regular blood glucose monitoring
Managed with tablets carrying hypoglycaemia risk (SU, glinides)	May drive and need not notify DVLA It is appropriate to offer SMBG at times relevant to driving to enable detection of hypoglycaemia May use CGM	May drive but <u>must</u> notify DVLA Regular SMBG—*at least twice daily* and at times relevant to driving (i.e. no more than 2 hours before the start of the first journey and every 2 hours whilst driving) Must use finger prick glucose testing
Insulin-treated	Blood glucose testing no more than 2 hours before the start of the first journey and every 2 hours while driving May use CGM	Regular blood glucose testing—at least twice daily, including on days when not driving and no more than 2 hours before the start of the first journey and every 2 hours whilst driving Must use finger prick glucose testing

NB more frequent self-monitoring may be required with any greater risk of hypoglycaemia (e.g. physical activity, altered meal routine).

DVLA, Driver and Vehicle Licensing Agency; DPP-4, dipeptidyl dipeptidase type 4; SGLT2, sodium–glucose cotransporter 2; GLP-1RA, glucagon-like peptide 1 receptor agonist; SU, sulfonylurea; SMBG, self-monitoring of blood glucose; CGM, continuous glucose monitoring.

purposes, unless there are concerns regarding their hypoglycaemia awareness.)
- The DVLA must also be notified if a person or their medical team feels they are at high risk of developing severe hypoglycaemia.

For group 2 drivers (bus/lorry)
- One episode of severe hypoglycaemia must be reported immediately, including sleep episodes.
- They must attend an annual review and present 3 months' worth of blood glucose readings (using a meter with memory function) by their usual doctor PLUS an annual review by an independent consultant diabetologist.

'Severe hypoglycaemia' is defined as hypoglycaemia requiring another person's assistance.

'Impaired awareness of hypoglycaemia' for group 1 drivers is defined as 'an inability to detect the onset of hypoglycaemia because of total absence of warning symptoms'.

Group 2 drivers must have full awareness of hypoglycaemia.

For group 1 drivers, interstitial glucose monitoring systems may be used for monitoring glucose at times relevant to driving, but users must also carry finger-prick capillary glucose testing equipment for driving and a finger-prick blood glucose reading MUST be taken in the following circumstances:
- When the glucose level is 4.0mmol/L or below
- When symptoms of hypoglycaemia are being experienced
- When the glucose monitoring system gives a reading that is not consistent with the symptoms being experienced (e.g. symptoms of hypoglycaemia are present, but the system reading does not indicate this).

For group 2 drivers, there is a legal requirement to monitor their blood glucose for the purpose of group 2 driving, and interstitial glucose monitoring systems are not permitted for the purposes of group 2 driving and licensing. Group 2 drivers who use these devices must continue to monitor finger-prick capillary blood glucose levels.

All drivers should be advised to:
- Carry a blood glucose meter and blood glucose strips in the car (in-date, not expired)
- Check blood glucose level before driving and on long journeys, and to stop every 2 hours to recheck
- Take a snack before driving if the blood glucose level is 5.0mmol/L or less
- Not drive if feeling hypoglycaemic or if the blood glucose level is <4.0mmol/L
- If hypoglycaemia develops whilst driving:
  - Stop the vehicle as soon as possible in a safe location.
  - Treat the hypoglycaemia and do not resume driving until 45 minutes after the blood glucose level has returned to normal (as it takes up to 45 minutes for the brain to recover fully).
- Always keep an emergency supply of fast-acting carbohydrate, such as glucose tablets or sweets, in the vehicle within easy reach of the driver.

- Take regular meals, snacks, and rest periods on long journeys, and always avoid alcohol.
- Declare they have diabetes when applying for motor insurance.

Reference

1. Driver and Vehicle Licensing Agency (2024). *Assessing fitness to drive—a guide for medical professionals.* Available at: ℘ https://assets.publishing.service.gov.uk/media/65cf7243e1bdec001a322 268/assessing-fitness-to-drive-february-2024.pdf

Sick day guidance

Intercurrent illness and infection in a person living with diabetes can escalate and result in more serious conditions, such as DKA, HHS, and/or acute kidney injury (AKI), which would require emergency hospital admission (see ➔ Chapter 12).

The aims of managing a person with diabetes during intercurrent illness are to:

- Manage blood glucose levels
- Ensure adequate calorie intake (consider meal replacements) and hydration with fluid replacement
- Test for, and manage (if present), ketones where relevant
- Recognize when further medical attention is required such as signs and symptoms of DKA/HSS or in special circumstances such as pregnancy.

NEVER stop insulin

Insulin doses may need to be ↑ during illness, especially if ketones are present (see ➔ Chapter 12 for suggested management of insulin during intercurrent illness).

Some medications need to be paused whilst a person is at risk of dehydration and restarted once eating and drinking normally again. These include:

- **S**odium–glucose cotransporter 2 inhibitors
- **A**ngiotensin-converting enzyme inhibitors[*]
- **D**iuretics[*]
- **M**etformin
- **A**ngiotensin receptor blockers[*]
- **N**on-steroidal anti-inflammatory medications.

([*] May need discussion with cardiology teams before pausing, e.g. in heart failure)

Further reading

Down S. How to advise on sick day rules. *Diabetes & Primary Care*. 2020;**22**:47–8. Available at: ℞ https://diabetesonthenet.com/diabetes-primary-care/how-to-advise-on-sick-day-rules/

Trend Diabetes (2022). *Type 1 diabetes: what to do when you are ill*. Available at: ℞ https://trenddiabetes.online/portfolio/type-1-diabetes-what-to-do-when-you-are-ill

Trend Diabetes (2022). *Type 2 diabetes: what to do when you are ill*. Available at: ℞ https://trenddiabetes.online/portfolio/type-2-diabetes-what-to-do-when-you-are-ill

Diabetes and cancer

It is estimated that 20% of people with cancer have concurrent diabetes.[1]

Individuals with a diagnosis of diabetes are at higher risk of developing several cancers, likely due to shared risk factors between the two conditions.

People with cancer are at ↑ risk of developing new-onset diabetes/hyperglycaemia, due to therapies which may be used in treatment pathways (e.g. steroids and immune checkpoint inhibitors). Such therapies and treatment will also cause a deterioration in glucose levels for anyone with pre-existing diabetes (see also ➲ Chapter 1).

People with cancer and diabetes are known to be at higher risk of developing infections and hospitalization, compared with those without diabetes, but also at risk of chemotherapy dose reductions and early treatment cessation.[2]

Several studies have demonstrated that hyperglycaemia is prognostic of worse overall survival and risk of cancer recurrence in a number of cancer subtypes.[2]

Symptoms of hyperglycaemia, in addition to cancer-specific and chemotherapy side effects, can be debilitating. This can have major negative impacts on diabetes self-care, including appetite, emotional well-being, access to diabetes care, and social impacts.

Collaboration between the oncology multidisciplinary team and the diabetes team is vital to ensure people receive appropriate and timely diabetes treatment, so to improve quality of life and reduce hospital admissions.

Optimal glycaemic levels during cancer treatment has significant implications for both cancer outcomes and survivorship.

Insulin therapy is often indicated and requires bespoke management.

For further information, including pathways for insulin management, see: Joint British Diabetes Societies for Inpatient Care (2021). *The management of glycaemic control in patients with cancer: guidance for the diabetes and oncology multidisciplinary teams.* Available at: ℘ https://abcd.care/sites/default/files/site_uploads/JBDS_Guidelines_Archive/JBDS_17_Oncology_Guideline_Final_21052021_Archive.pdf

References

1. Joint British Diabetes Societies for Inpatient Care (2021). *The management of glycaemic control in patients with cancer: guidance for the diabetes and oncology multidisciplinary teams.* Available at: ℘ https://abcd.care/sites/default/files/site_uploads/JBDS_Guidelines_Archive/JBDS_17_Oncology_Guideline_Final_21052021_Archive.pdf
2. Joharatnam-Hogan N, Carter TJ, Reynolds N, Ho JH, Adam S, Board R (last updated 2021). Diabetes mellitus in people with cancer. In: Feingold KR, Anawalt B, Blackman MR, *et al.* (editors). *Endotext* [Internet]. South Dartmouth, MA: MDText.com Inc. Available at: ℘ www.ncbi.nlm.nih.gov/books/NBK575925

Chapter 18

Diabetes care delivery

Introduction

Throughout the chapters of the book, the authors have defined gold standards for diabetes care.

In the post-coronavirus disease 2019 (COVID-19) era, individual health care professionals, teams, systems, and wider organizations face multiple challenges in striving to ensure equitable, holistic, and optimal care for all persons living with diabetes.

Challenges include:
- Increasing numbers of people being diagnosed with diabetes
- Workforce capacity
- Variability in workforce knowledge and skills
- Financial pressures
- Increasing numbers of people with early-onset type 2 diabetes (T2D)
- An ageing population with multiple long-term conditions
- Lack of appropriate care pathways
- Variability in access to care
- Health inequalities.

This chapter will look to highlight best-practice models of integrated and inpatient hospital diabetes care, how to ensure appropriate diabetes nursing standards so to make sure that the 'right person is seen at the right time, in the right place by the right health care professional/team'.

The chapter will also discuss how we can better reach and care for our hardly reached populations who are living with diabetes.

Models of care

For all care models, it is important to consider co-design and collaboration with people living with diabetes, all health care professionals, commissioners, and allied professionals.

Key components for successful coordinated diabetes care are illustrated in Fig. 18.1, with evaluation and audit as essential for ongoing optimal care.[1]

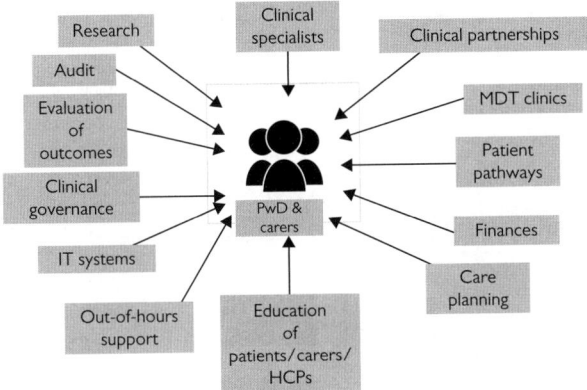

Fig. 18.1 Key ingredients for optimal coordinated diabetes care.

Reference

1. Ali SN, Alicea S, Avery L, Beba H, Kanumilli N, Milne N. (2001). *Best Practice in the Delivery of Diabetes Care in the Primary Care Network.* Available at: ℘ https://diabetes-resources-pro duction.s3.eu-west-1.amazonaws.com/resources-s3/public/2021-04/Diabetes-in-the-Primary-Care-Network-Structure-April-2021_with-logos.pdf

Integrated care

For optimal outcomes in diabetes, there is a pressing need to effectively facilitate and support the flow of people with diabetes through the different areas of the National Health Service (NHS) and wider social support services, depending on their needs at the point of health care access.

Diabetes Support Team model of care

The formation and emergence of primary care networks (PCNs) have afforded the opportunity to strengthen integration between primary, community, and specialist care, and to provide diabetes services that address the needs of the person with diabetes, including the specific needs of underserved populations.

The document 'Best Practice in the Delivery of Diabetes Care in the Primary Care Network Structure'[1] advocates for a four-tier approach to diabetes care surrounded by allied support services such as remission programmes for T2D, mental health services, and social prescribing initiatives, as illustrated in Fig. 18.2.

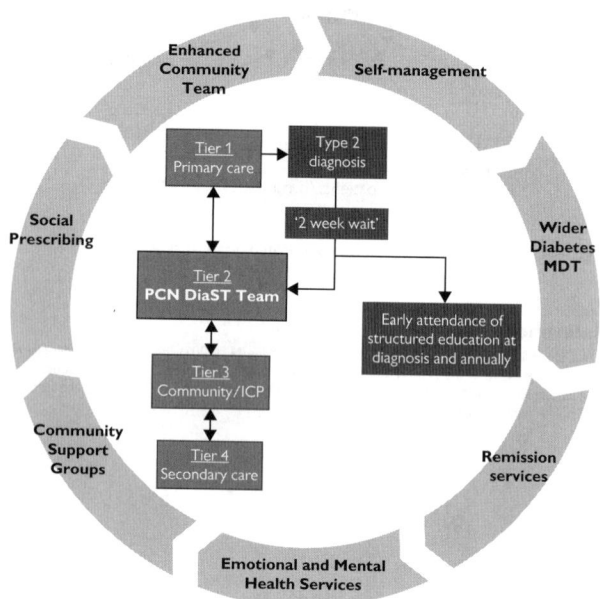

Fig. 18.2 Diabetes Support Team (DiaST) model of care.

Seamless movement of people living with diabetes through
the tiers dependent on needs

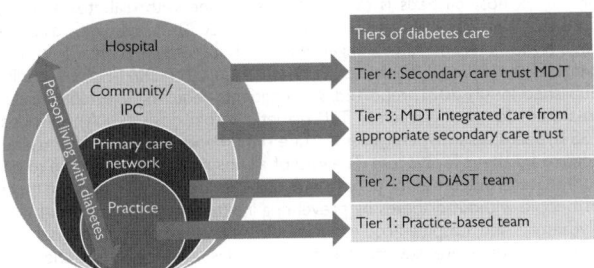

Fig. 18.3 Seamless movement of people living with diabetes through the tiers dependent on needs.

The authors of the PCN document advocate for a Diabetes Support Team (DiaST)/lead across PCNs to provide for:
- Early referral to diabetes education and/or remission of T2D programmes where relevant
- Direct care for persons with more complex diabetes care needs
- Diabetes-related clinical governance, education, and mentorship for all health care professionals within the PCN
- Outreach to underserved populations
- Communication/link with community and secondary care services.

This pathway provides for the seamless movement of persons with diabetes through the tiers dependent on needs, whilst ensuring health care professionals feel supported and empowered in diabetes care (see Fig. 18.3).

Tiers 3 and 4 would be persons requiring specialist/consultant input, as advocated for in the 'Portsmouth Super Six Model of Care',[2] including:
- Inpatient diabetes
- Antenatal diabetes
- Diabetes foot care
- Diabetes nephropathy (dialysis or progressive decline of renal function)
- Insulin pumps/hybrid closed loop
- Young onset T2D (including children).

References

1. Ali SN, Alicea S, Avery L, Beba H, Kanumilli N, Milne N. (2001). *Best Practice in the Delivery of Diabetes Care in the Primary Care Network.* Available at: ℜ https://diabetes-resources-production.s3.eu-west-1.amazonaws.com/resources-s3/public/2021-04/Diabetes-in-the-Primary-Care-Network-Structure-April-2021_with-logos.pdf
2. Kar P. The Super Six model: integrating diabetes care across Portsmouth and south-east Hampshire. *Diabetes & Primary Care.* 2012;**14**(5):277–83. Available at: ℜ https://diabetesonthenet.com/wp-content/uploads/dpc14-5-277-83-1.pdf

A good inpatient diabetes service

Inpatient care for diabetes costs the NHS £2.5 billion per year. Currently, one in six hospital beds is occupied by someone with diabetes and it is predicted that this will rise to one in four by 2030. People with diabetes have higher infection rates, longer lengths of stay, and ↑ mortality in hospitals. The National Diabetes Inpatient Audit (NaDIA)-Harms audit,[1] published in July 2021, reported 3200 patients requiring injectable rescue treatment for hypoglycaemia, 750 diabetic ketoacidosis (DKA) episodes, 135 hyperosmolar hyperglycaemic state (HHS) episodes, and 515 hospital-acquired diabetic foot ulcers. The goal of all hospital trusts should be to ensure that the outcomes for people with diabetes are no different from those of people without diabetes by preventing inpatient hyperglycaemia, hypoglycaemia, and hospital-acquired foot ulcers and ensuring safe discharge planning. There are several recommendations available from the Joint British Diabetes Societies (JBDS), Diabetes UK, and the Getting It Right First Time (GIRFT) team. The JBDS has implemented high-quality evidence-based guidelines and inpatient care pathways to improve inpatient diabetes care across the UK. The GIRFT programme aims to bring high-quality care in hospitals by reducing unwanted variations in services and practices.

There are several recommendations available from JBDS, Diabetes UK, and the GIRFT team such as:
- Multidisciplinary diabetes inpatient teams that are available 7 days a week
- Strong clinical leadership from diabetes inpatient teams
- Mandatory diabetes training for all health care professionals
- Better support in hospitals for people with diabetes to take ownership of their diabetes
- Effective hospital systems to identify people with diabetes on admission to hospital and to monitor those at risk throughout their stay
- All hospitals to have processes in place to make sure mistakes are owned, understood, and managed by the clinical teams involved.

The Diabetes Care Accreditation Programme (DCAP), set up by the Royal College of Physicians and Diabetes UK, also aims to improve inpatient diabetes care by setting quality standards and measuring service performance through external peer assessment.

Reference

1. NHS England (2021). National Diabetes Inpatient Audit—Harms 2020 England. Available at: ⅏ https://digital.nhs.uk/data-and-information/publications/statistical/national-diabetes-inpatient-audit---harms/national-diabetes-inpatient-audit---harms-2020

Further reading

Joint British Diabetes Societies (2019). *A good inpatient diabetes service*. Available at: ⅏ https://abcd.care/sites/default/files/site_uploads/JBDS_Guidelines_Current/JBDS_14_A_Good_Inpatient_Service_Updated_060720.pdf

Diabetes UK (2018). *Making hospitals safe for people with diabetes*. Available at: ⅏ www.diabetes.org.uk/resources-s3/2018-12/Making%20Hospitals%20safe%20for%20people%20with%20diabetes_FINAL%20%28002%29.pdf

Multidisciplinary teams and care

Multidisciplinary working brings together relevant health care professionals and services in supporting best-practice diabetes care.

As we continue to move towards holistic multimorbidity care, rather than a blinkered 'glucocentric' approach, in diabetes, it is vital that we co-design services and work together for the best interest of the person with diabetes.

Each team member can enhance care and provide support, depending on a person's needs and complexity.

Fig. 18.4 illustrates an example of a modern diabetes team, including the use of technology/IT systems. It is important that we recognize, communicate, and involve relevant team members.

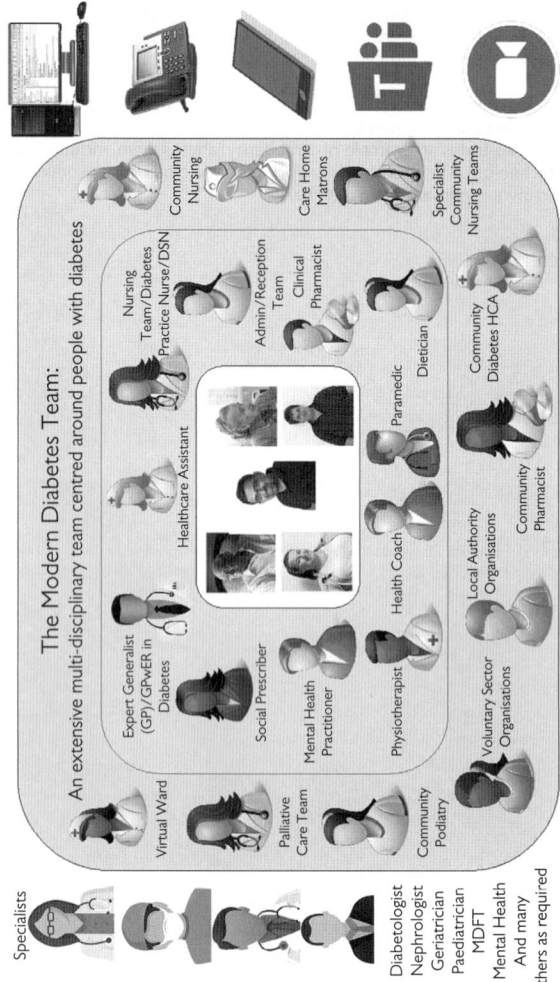

Fig. 18.4 The modern diabetes team: an extensive multidisciplinary team centred around people with diabetes.

Reproduced here with the kind permission of Professor Clare Hambling, National Clinical Director, Diabetes & Obesity NHS England.

Tackling health inequalities

NHS England defines health inequalities as unfair and avoidable differences in health across the population and between different groups within society.

Research and national data have repeatedly shown that people from black and South Asian communities and people living in deprivation are more likely to develop T2D but are less likely to be able to access the care, treatments, and guidance they need. In T1D, persons from the same cohorts are less likely to receive the care they need, including access to technology.

In considering the determinants of good health, it is important to consider the infrastructures and requirements that surround a person, as illustrated in Fig. 18.5. It is relevant that we consider wider population health initiatives and council planning.

The 'Build Back Fairer in Greater Manchester: Health Equity and Dignified Lives' by the Institute of Health Equity gives further learnings on how the wider society and environment impact health. Applicable to other areas of the country, the report is available at: ℅ www.instituteofhealthequity.org/resources-reports/build-back-fairer-in-greater-manchester-health-equity-and-dignified-lives/build-back-fairer-in-greater-manchester-main-report.pdf

In 2023, Diabetes UK launched the Tackling Inequality Commission, inviting people living with, and at risk of, diabetes who are most affected by health inequalities and those working closest to health inequality to share their experiences and look to solutions in narrowing/eliminating the gap. The findings of the report, including suggestions for 'levelling up' are available at: ℅ https://diabetes-resources-production.s3.eu-west-1.amazonaws.com/resources-s3/public/2023-11/366_Tackling_Inequality_Commission_Report_DIGITAL%20(1).pdf

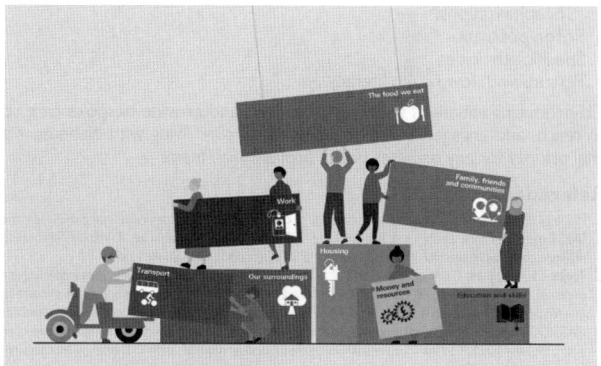

Fig. 18.5 'What Builds Good health'

Available at ℅ https://www.health.org.uk/news-and-comment/charts-and-infographics/what-builds-good-health

Underserved populations

An important aspect in reducing health inequalities is for diabetes teams, PCNs, and Integrated Care Boards (ICBs) to look to whom they are not engaging with/hardly reaching for diabetes care. Data show that persons not receiving their diabetes care processes (see ⮕ Chapter 9) each year are those more likely to have poorer health outcomes, including higher morbidity and mortality from the virus during the COVID-19 pandemic.

Such cohorts that practices might not be reaching include:

- Persons living with higher levels of deprivation
- Working age groups[1]
- Persons with a learning disability.
  - People with a learning difficulty are 2–3 times more likely to develop either T1D or T2D. For T2D, it is more likely to develop at an earlier age than would normally be expected.
  - The 'International Consensus Guidelines: Reasonable Adjustments in the Management of Type 2 Diabetes in Adults with Intellectual and Developmental Disabilities'[2] provides a wealth of information relating to appropriate, reasonable adjustments to enable safe and effective care where there may be challenges in accessing education/care and safe insulin use.
- Persons with severe mental health illness (SMI), including those in mental health care facilities:
  - Diabetes is 2–3 times more prevalent in people with SMI. Among people with diabetes, people with a history of SMI have poorer cardiovascular and mortality outcomes.[3]
- Persons who are homeless:
  - T2D is notably more prevalent among homeless individuals, and challenges relating to inadequate nutrition, risk of violence, potential comorbidities, and poor access to routine health care lead to higher rates of diabetes-related emergency department visits and hospitalizations.[4]
- Prison population[5]
- Specific ethnicities
- Persons with low health literacy.

Co-producing initiatives to identify, support, and provide bespoke care so to reach, and engage with, all cohorts of persons living with diabetes is a vital priority for any diabetes health professional/team.

References

1. Milne N. Engaging with and optimising care for people under age 50 years with type 2 diabetes: the DiaST model of care. *Diabetes & Primary Care*. 2023;**25**(6):193. Available at: ⬤ https://diabeteso nthenet.com/wp-content/uploads/4.-Milne_EOT2D-service-evaluation-1.pdf
2. Taggart L, Tripp H, Conder J, *et al.* (2021). *International consensus guidelines: reasonable adjustments in the management of type 2 diabetes in adults with intellectual & developmental disabilities.* International Association for the Scientific Study of Intellectual & Developmental Disabilities (IASSIDD): Health Special Interest Research Group. Available at: ⬤ www.iassidd.org/wp-cont ent/uploads/2021/05/Int-Consensus-Guidelines-Management-of-Type-2-Diabetes-Intellectual-Disabiliteis-IASSIDD-Taggart-et-al.-2021.pdf
3. Fleetwood KJ, Wild SH, Licence KAM, Mercer SW, Smith DJ, Jackson CA; Scottish Diabetes Research Network Epidemiology Group. Severe mental illness and type 2 diabetes outcomes and

complications: a nationwide cohort study. *Diabetes Care*. 2023;**46**(7):1363–71. Available at: ℘ https://doi.org/10.2337/dc23-0177

4. Benz F. Type 2 diabetes management in the homeless population: health inequality and the Housing First approach. *British Journal of Diabetes*. 2023;**23**:69–76. Available at: ℘ https://bjd-abcd.com/index.php/bjd/article/view/1131

5. Mills LS. Diabetes behind bars: considerations for managing diabetes within the prison setting. *Diabetes & Primary Care*. 2015;**17**:290–5 Available at: ℘ https://diabetesonthenet.com/diabe tes-primary-care/diabetes-behind-bars-considerations-for-managing-diabetes-within-the-prison-setting-and-after-release

Nursing competencies

'An Integrated Career and Competency Framework for Adult Diabetes Nursing'[1] is an integral tool for identifying the educational needs and competency levels of nurses and unregistered practitioners.

It covers 28 topic areas, ranging from screening and early diagnosis of T2D through to caring for someone with diabetes at the end of their life, with recommended competencies grouped at five levels:

- Unregistered practitioner
- Competent nurse
- Experienced or proficient nurse
- Senior practitioner or expert nurse
- Nurse consultant.

Users of the framework should identify their level of practice (or level to which they aspire) and the topics relevant to their area of practice. The framework also includes useful resources to signpost users to build knowledge, with a few examples of tools which could be used to assess competence.

NB as this book goes to print, an update to this competency framework is expected.

Reference

1. Trend Diabetes (2021). *An integrated career and competency framework for adult diabetes nursing*. Available at: ℘ https://trenddiabetes.online/wp-content/uploads/2020/04/Framework_6th_EDN_TREND_FINAL.pdf

Organizations supporting diabetes care

- Diabetes UK. Available at: ℘ www.diabetes.org.uk (all types of diabetes).
- Breakthrough T1D and Available at: ℘ https://breakthrought1d.org.uk (more bespoke for type 1 diabetes).
- Primary Care Diabetes and Obesity Society. Available at: ℘ https://www.pcdosociety.org/
- Diabetes Specialist Nurse Forum UK. Available at: ℘ www.diabetesspecialistnurseforumuk.co.uk
- Diabetes Inpatient Specialist Nurse Forum Group. Available at: ℘ www.disn-uk.co.uk
- The Association of British Clinical Diabetologists. Available at: ℘ https://abcd.care
- Joint British Diabetes Societies (JBDS) for Inpatient Care Group. Available at: ℘ https://abcd.care/jbds-ip
- Welsh Academy for Nursing in Diabetes (WAND). Available at: ℘ www.wand-wales.co.uk/education
- TREND Diabetes. Available at: ℘ https://trenddiabetes.online
- EDEN Diabetes. Available at: ℘ www.edendiabetes.com
- Diabetes Psychology Network. Available at: ℘ https://diabetespsychologymatters.com
- The ABCD Diabetes Technology Network. Available at: ℘ https://abcd.care/abcd-diabetes-technology-network
- American Diabetes Association. Available at: ℘ https://diabetes.org
- Foundation of European Nurses in Diabetes (FEND). Available at: ℘ www.fend.org
- European Association for the Study of Diabetes. Available at: ℘ www.easd.org/index.html
- International Diabetes Federation. Available at: ℘ https://idf.org
- World Health Organization. Available at: ℘ www.who.int

Index

For the benefit of digital users, indexed terms that span two pages (e.g., 52–53) may, on occasion, appear on only one of those pages.

Tables, figures, and boxes are indicated by an italic *t*, *f*, and *b* following the page/paragraph number.